FROM PAIN TO PEACE WITH ENDO

Lessons Learned on the Road to Healing Endometriosis

Aubree Deimler

From Pain to Peace with Endo:
Lessons Learned on the Road to Healing Endometriosis
Copyright© 2014 by Aubree Deimler

The information presented herein is not medical advice
and is not intended to diagnose, treat, cure, or prevent any disease and
should not in any way be used as a substitute for the advice of a physician,
therapist, or other licensed healthcare practitioner. The content of this book
is for general instruction only. Each person's physical, emotional,
and spiritual condition is unique. Please consult your doctor for matters
pertaining to your specific health and diet.

To contact the author, visit
www.peacewithendo.com
Cover art by: Teddi Black
ISBN-13: 978-0692297827
ISBN-10: 0692297820

Printed in the United States of America

Dedication

I dedicate this book to all my fellow endo warriors, who struggle with the physical and emotional pain from endometriosis.

This book is for those who long for relief and those open to discovery into the realms of possibility, the possibility of finding healing. And peace with endo.

I extend these words to you with hope.

Contents

Preface

When I was first diagnosed with endometriosis, I had so many questions. My intuition told me not to take the hormone-altering drugs offered to me, and when my body ached after laparoscopic surgery, I told myself that I did not want to do that again. I was overwhelmed and felt so alone.

Despite what seemed to be a dismal diagnosis, an inner voice whispered that I could not give up hope. So with continued faith in the power of the body to heal, I paved a new way. I researched, experimented, and developed a true passion for whole, natural healing.

This book includes the lessons that I learned on my journey to healing endometriosis, things I wish I'd known from the start.

It also includes my very personal story, which I haven't shared with many. An introvert by nature, I've been known throughout my life as the quiet girl. I found, however, that during those times when I did share my story, a great healing opened up for me.

When I spoke up about endometriosis, it connected me with other women who had it too. In most circumstances, these were also women who did not make a habit of talking about this silent condition.

There is nothing greater than finding someone else who understands the pain associated with this condition, which strikes at the very center of our womanhood.

The women that I've met with endometriosis are some of the most caring and supportive I've ever known. For with pain comes compassion and gratitude for the little things.

By sharing my story and knowledge gained, it is these women that I hope to help.

Falling into a place of chronic pain made me search for something more. When we hit the bottom, there is only one way to go—up. That road led me to finding peace with endometriosis.

I hope that by sharing my story and the lessons I picked up along that way, I am able to help you get there as well.

To connect with me further please visit www.peacewithendo.com.

Acknowledgements

As my passion for health and wellness grew, I really wanted to share all this valuable information that made such a significant impact in my life. Since I was a little girl it has been a dream of mine to write and publish a book.

I'm not sure that this collection of lessons would have made it through the publication process and into your hands without the motivation, passion, and direction that I gained from my writing coaches: author and speaker, Lindsey "The Food Mood Girl" Smith, and Joshua Rosenthal, an amazing, inspiring coach and founder of the Institute for Integrative Nutrition (IIN), the school that changed my life.

Thank you for helping me through this process and making this dream a reality.

I want to thank my full time coach and husband, Ryan, for his support along this journey. When I wanted to quit, he was there to push me back up. His positive words and motivation really helped me when I had doubts about my writing and me.

I extend sincere gratitude to the beautiful, kind women with endometriosis who have truly touched my life. I want to thank those of you who are passionate about health and wellness and who share this information with others. I have learned so much about this condition and the direction to take to overcome it with the priceless knowledge and support of my fellow endo sisters.

There is a lot that goes into publication after the writing is done. I am proud to say that fellow endo warriors touched many of the pieces of this book.

I extend great gratitude to my editors, Leah Campbell, who helped bring my thoughts in order and encouraged me to share more of my story and Kathy Tracy who helped improve the flow of my words.

I send further gratitude to my photographer, Audrey Michel, who not only took beautiful pictures of me, but also supported my journey of writing.

I extend gratitude to Amanda MacCabe for beautifully laying out the interior. I will always remember how excited I was to see my words laid out like a book!

I extend additional gratitude towards my cover and designer, Teddi Black. Thank you for beautifully wrapping up my collection of words.

TO BLEED,
TO LOVE,
TO LOSE

"Sometimes it's worth lingering on the journey for a while before getting to the destination."

~ Richelle Mead, The Indigo Spell

MEET YOUR AUNT FLOW

When I was 11 years old my mother sat me down to have a talk. She told me a little bit about how things worked in a woman's menstrual cycle, explaining that soon I should be expecting a visit from my little monthly friend.

That conversation freaked me out.

"That's not going to happen for awhile though, right?" I asked.

"Sooner than not, my dear," my mother replied.

She was right. My period showed not too long after that conversation and it was much more than I anticipated. Things went very wrong from the start. My whole body hurt; excruciating pain radiated from my very center, leaving me breathless and bedridden.

My mother rubbed my aching legs as I lay halfway up in the bed, a heating pad clutched to my abdomen. She put a cool washcloth on my face, but this just aggravated me. The pain was horrible, pulsing from my uterus. I could tell by the look on her face that she wanted so badly to help me, but she didn't know what to do. And there really wasn't anything she *could* do. Nothing stopped the pain.

I went to see a male family doctor. As a young and timid girl, I struggled to describe to this man the pain I was experiencing with my periods. My voice shook, barely audible. He looked halfway interested then wrote me a prescription for ibuprofen before sending me on my way.

The pain with my periods continued to torment me, keeping me in bed for days each month away from school, away from work. Life passed by outside my window as I curled into a ball, suffocated by pure agony. I complained about the menstrual pain to my gynecologists for years to come, but they all told me the same thing: take ibuprofen...take a *higher* dose of ibuprofen.

Nobody really listened. They just continued to tell me to pop those little over-the-counter pain pills. So I did—all the time—even though they gave me a stomach ache. It reached a point where I had to make the choice: stomach ache or pain? I almost always chose the stomach ache.

As the pain progressed, I didn't know what to do. It was disrupting my life. When I was 17 I told my mother that I was going to see another doctor. She guessed they might prescribe me birth control for the pain. She was right. The doctor, this time a female, also wrote a script for high-strength ibuprofen (of course).

I took the suggestion and started on birth control. Immediately I got very sick with daily nausea, dizziness, and headaches. I went back to the doctor and was prescribed various brands before finally settling on the lowest dose estrogen pill. Even then I was still terribly nauseous and my mood swings continued to accelerate. But those little white pills really helped the menstrual pain so I stayed on them. It would be a decade before I stopped taking them.

SEARCHING FOR LOVE

When I was 15 those magical words first slipped out of my lips: "I think I love him." My girlfriends swooned when I said it.

Growing into a young woman, I think I had some skewed perceptions about this notion of love, having fallen prey to scenes in movies and on TV. But regardless, I was in love. He was tall and could drive! Older and with his life planned out, he was training to take a position with the Air Force Academy.

As our relationship progressed over time, things heated up. This was the first time I really started to experience the pain *down there* outside of my period. I flinched almost every time he touched me. I was a virgin and very young so I was ill equipped to truly evaluate whether or not this was normal.

For Valentine's Day he presented me with a signature pink and white-striped box. Opening it I found a lacy, crème-colored lingerie set. When I lifted it up to look at it, my eyes fixated on what was beneath: a box of Trojan condoms. My jaw dropped. His message was clear.

"I want to see you in that," he said.

My face was beet red as I quickly shut the box. After an awkward moment, I excused myself. When I went home, I flipped through the pamphlet that came in the condom box and my stomach turned. I wasn't ready for this.

But I loved him, right?

In the face of such a big step, I wasn't sure. A short time after that, I was given the news: he was seeing someone else behind my back. My young teenage heart broke and I fell into a world of tears and disregard. I turned somewhat violent against myself; I obviously wasn't worth his love.

I drowned my sorrows in alcohol and rebellious behavior. This included an illegal, underage tattoo—an outline of a dragon that turned out looking more like a sad little lizard on my upper right shoulder. The cut of the tattoo gun was satisfying on my skin.

Following this came rounds of piercings in all sorts of places that shouldn't be pierced. I also dabbled in some drugs, anything that took my mind out of my physical body, the body that I didn't really care about anymore.

My self-esteem was very low. I bounced in and out of different relationships, seeking the missing piece: love. But the pressure to have sex always seemed to present itself instead. I was very well-endowed and had a slim waist, and while I didn't know it at the time, I was beautiful. The guys in my life were interested in my physical appearance and the pressure mounted—literally.

When I was 17, I got into another not-so-great relationship that revolved around drugs and alcohol. One night, as we downed shots of hard alcohol, things got heated physically. Before I knew it, I was in his bed and he was on top of me and extremely persistent about his intentions. I tried to move but his arms were tight on each side of my shoulders. Pinned. I was afraid and far from ready. And this was surely not love. The pressure and my fear reflected down there, where he forced his way in.

He promised me a bottle of vodka when it was done.

Afterward I was alone in the bathroom and saw gobs of blood on the toilet paper and a felt sharp pain between my legs. My innocence was gone and the pain was real, radiating from my center to my toes.

NO ONE WILL EVER LOVE YOU

From there I moved into yet another unhealthy relationship that included quite a bit of verbal abuse. I witnessed firsthand the effects of a family torn by alcoholism and the importance of a father's behavior on his son.

The drugs and alcohol continued for me as well as I tried to feed an undeniable desire to escape my skin, my being. I was very unhappy, but I believed a part of me felt that this was what I was worth. I recalled a few of the last words he spat at me as our relationship neared the end: "No one will *ever* love you."

Those words stuck with me and took shelter in the darkest recesses of my mind, finding presence at opportune moments. I struggled for years with depression, a deep bleakness that kept me in bed for days at a time, flooding tears and emotion so deep inside of me. These emotions were based on the notion that nobody loved me. There was one particular instance where this pain drove me to take as many pill bottles as I could carry from the medicine cabinet. I returned to my bed and laid the bottles in a circle around me.

I sat in the middle of them contemplating that resounding thought of dis-love. I had thoughts of swallowing as many pills as I could so that I could drift into a never-ending sleep. I didn't want to *be* anymore. I was tired of my existence. Nobody would care if I were gone. I was unloved.

Fortunately, there was a knock at my door and my brother walked in. This shocked me back into reality.

The thought of suicide didn't leave my mind for many years to come. There were periods when the emotional pain was so excruciating that I fantasized about literally cutting the pain out of me. While I never did, I can definitely relate to those who do this.

I did get a couple more tattoos—perhaps the more socially accepted way to cut—leaving behind a mark of the time.

DATE TO REMEMBER

When I was 20 I moved out of my parents' house into an apartment with a gal that I worked with. My new roommate watched as my lingering depression kept me cooped up for hours in my bedroom. When I did leave, it was often with tear-streaked cheeks.

One day she suggested that I meet a friend of hers who was single. Still broken-hearted from years of abuse, I shrugged it off as a whatever. A few days later I received a voicemail on my phone. It was from my roommate's friend Jeff, wondering if I wanted to connect with him. He left his name and number, and then I heard a beep in the message—the sound of another call coming in. Instead of successfully clicking over to the other call he remained on my line, my voicemail recording his every word.

"I'm on the phone with this really hot girl—"

At that point he realized he was still being recorded on my line and after letting out few expletives and laughter, the message ended.

I smiled and tossed aside my phone, with little intention of calling him back. As I turned to walk out of the room, the phone rang. I picked it up and it was Jeff. I had to give him some props for calling back after his amusing mishap and gave him yet another chance to chat further over dinner. We planned it for a couple of nights later during my work break.

I was very nervous. I'd never been on a blind date before. When he walked in, I was pleasantly surprised. He had a cute, crooked grin and the workings of a slight Southern accent. His skin was tan and his shoulders broad and strong.

We hit it off over dinner, sharing bouts of laughter. His manners were very polite, a quality I surely recognized. I ate very little; my stomach was still in nervous knots. I'm sure my face was a crimson color the whole time. He dropped me back at work and we parted ways. I was left with memories of his smile and butterflies in my stomach.

I couldn't wait to see him again.

Things moved pretty quickly after our initial meeting. We spent a lot of time together and for the first time in a long time, I allowed my broken heart to open again with possibility. This man walked into my life and made me feel loved. He talked highly of me to his friends and family and was sure to express his gratitude for having me in his life.

Things weren't always sweetness and roses; we struggled for sure, but through it all I found a connection that I hadn't previously believed was possible. My thoughts of never being loved faded. This belief was solidified one night when among a group of his good friends he knelt before me and held out a ring. My head swirled when he placed it on my finger. I was only 21 years old and honestly a little unsure about marriage.

Was this really happening?

A short while later, as I tried on wedding dresses with my mother, reality sunk in: this was really happening. I sought out big cathedral churches for our wedding with visions of me walking down the aisle to be greeted by an eternal love.

A NOT SO HAPPY ENDING

Unfortunately, this love story stopped short one sunny afternoon in October. I was napping on the couch after attending a long day of college classes and woke to a knock at the door. I got up, still half asleep, and through the peephole I spotted a police officer and another woman dressed in a suit. With nervous waves of energy rushing through me, I opened up the door.

The woman asked if I knew Jeff and asked what our relationship was. When I told her, she asked if she could come in. I stepped aside so they could pass and tried to stifle the shake rattling inside my gut. Jeff had been in a car accident.

"Is he okay?" I asked.

"He didn't survive."

She went on to explain how he had died on or shortly after impact and likely didn't feel any pain. By the time the paramedics arrived, shortly after the crash, he had already passed on. Much of what she said after those words was mute to me. I went into a shocked state, unable to comprehend reality. It was as if a loud hum filled my brain. A painful ache radiated from my chest.

In a daze, I walked past the woman as she was midsentence and into the hall. I think I managed to mumble an, "Excuse me. I'll be right back."

Some type of gravitational pull led me to my neighbor Ryan's apartment, which was caddy corner to mine. I knocked on the door and he answered. I think he could tell something was wrong from my white-as-a-ghost face and trembling hands. My voice shook as I told him the news. I felt completely out of my body, as if I was look-ing down on the scene happening around me. It all felt like a dream.

Ryan was a good friend of Jeff's. His face dropped when he heard my words, the words that I needed for him to tell me were true. I needed confirmation that this was really happening. He shut the door to his apartment and came with me back to mine, somehow willing to confirm this new reality even as he himself was grieving.

SEEKING ANSWERS FROM THE SKY

The following day I went to church with my parents. This was my first time back in five years or so. Grief stricken, I went in hopes that it would somehow help.

I walked numbly into the church. The air inside was cool and smelled familiar, a mix of incense and burning candles. I followed my mother into the worship area and watched her tip her fingers into the well of holy water and make the sign of the cross. I followed her down the center aisle, light streaming in through a long line of stained glass windows. I don't remember much after that, besides the automatic sitting, standing, and chanting ingrained into my subconscious from a very young age. Even though it had been years since I'd gone to mass, I remembered all the steps.

There was a large statue of Mother Mary. I looked at her sad face for a long while. I felt as though it was a reflection of me. My parents suggested that I speak with a priest, hoping that would somehow mend my overflowing grief, my broken heart.

The priest took me back to his chambers and I sat on a plaid flannel couch. He sat across from me in a wicker chair. Not much was spoken. An eerie kind of silence hung that made the hairs on my arms stand straight up. He said a prayer for Jeff's saved soul and for me.

I walked out of the church that day and did not return again for many years. After the death of someone so close, I had sought out solace and hope for something more than my physical reality. I wanted to believe that his soul was safe, at peace. But I did not find my solace there.

Taking Shelter Next Door

I didn't want to be in my apartment anymore. It was so cold there, so empty without Jeff. I spent the next couple of days cleaning out all his clothes from the closet where his smell lingered. I felt better once his stuff was gone; looking at it had made it easy to think he might return.

Instead of fighting my existence in the void of my apartment, my presence shifted over to Ryan's place. We'd hung out nearly every day since the dreadful knock on my door. He let me crash on his futon after having several panic attacks about being alone in the confines of my dark bedroom.

I crossed my legs underneath me on the couch and listened to Ryan pluck on the strings of his guitar. I sipped on a glass of wine and relished his company. He helped me to not lose my smile and was there to listen to my thoughts on the subject of death and lost love.

He told me that Jeff lied to me about quitting smoking. That he sneaked over to his apartment on frequent occasions and smoked three or four cigarettes before filling his mouth with mints to cover it up from me. All I could do was laugh.

After setting down his guitar, he tossed me over a gaming controller. "Want to play?" he smiled.

I tried to smile back, "Sure."

We dueled each other in a fighting video game where the women fighters had grossly oversized breasts and the men had overstated muscles. We laughed as the boobs bobbed up and down in dramatic fashion. The wine helped the giggles to continue well into the night.

Rooted in the mutual loss of someone we both loved, my relationship with Ryan provided me with a sliver of stability and the hope that there was life after loss.

SHEEP ON THE MOUNTAIN

Once morning broke and I had to return to my cold apartment, reality reared its ugly head again. I was alone...sort of. I still felt Jeff's presence there. It was hard to believe that I would never see him again.

I could only tolerate a certain amount of time in my apartment before I had to get out. I grabbed my bike and struggled to get it off the patio and out the front door. Carrying it down three flights of stairs I realized how heavy it was and stopped several times to rest. Jeff always carried the bikes down the stairs. The thought shot a pang through my heart.

I managed to make it down without dropping the bike or seriously injuring myself and then tried to attach the bike rack's straps on the back of my Civic. Jeff had always done this and I had no idea how to do it myself. Eventually, I tossed the straps aside in frustration.

Ryan pulled in a couple spots away and approached me with a smile. "Need some help?"

He hooked up the rack and lifted my bike onto it. "Going for a ride?" he asked.

"Yes," I said, wishing that I'd known he was going to be home. I may have chosen differently.

He double-checked to make sure the straps around the bike were secure, "Have a good time," he said before he walked away.

I drove in silence up to a bike path where Jeff and I often rode together. I pumped my legs as I moved the bike up the path, happy to be outside. It was a warm October day, broken up by bursts of cooling wind.

A short distance up the path, the trail began to run parallel to a roaring river. The sound of the water sang in rhythm with my breath and the steady circle of my legs that propelled me forward. I lifted my thighs off the seat as the incline picked up. I always struggled with this part.

You can do it.

The reminder of Jeff's voice sounded in my mind. I pumped my legs harder as sweat poured down my face.

When I hit the top of the hill, I pulled my bike over to a rest stop that included a couple of picnic tables beneath a wooden covering. Jeff and I had stopped there many times. I leaned my bike against one of the picnic tables and sat on top of it.

I watched the water flow down the river in bubbling ripples of movement. It never stopped. I felt closest to Jeff when I was out in the beautiful world, soaking in the simple realities of nature. I felt him through the warm sunlight and in a subtle breeze that kicked up fallen leaves. I looked up at the blue sky with billowing white clouds and whispered a soft prayer; a soft message to my lost love and the energy source that held him now. I regained a sense of control by saying these prayers in the sanctuary of nature. I surrendered the things out of my control.

As I got up to leave my spot by the river, I spotted the carving of our initials in one of the wooden canopy's posts. I ran my fingertips atop the indention and tears trickled down my cheeks.

Riding down the hill was a nice break for my tired legs. I gently pumped the brake when I felt out of control, but for the most part I let momentum pull me forward and fought through the fear of going too fast. As I turned a bend in the path, a memory surfaced. On one of Jeff's solo trips up this same path he had been chased down the hill by a bighorn sheep. He told the story about it often and was so animated during his recollection of the events.

As I flew down the hill, I couldn't help but smile. I imagined how I would feel if I was being chased by a bighorn sheep. I think I laughed out loud.

When I reached the bottom of the hill I came across a man walking solo on the other side of the path. He had a big white beard and mustache and a powerful disposition about him. He sort of glided up the path, in no hurry, enjoying his time amidst the beautiful nature.

When I passed him he greeted me with a big smile, "See any sheep up on the mountain today?" he asked.

"No, not today," I replied and broke out into a big grin.

In that moment I understood that there was something more. On that beautiful October day I recognized the message from something higher that things were all right. The love that I lost stayed with me in a spiritual sense, in small beautiful messages like the white bearded man strolling along the path.

PICKING AND PROBING

Into my early twenties, my life included a lot more trips to the gynecologist, especially after having a pap smear come back abnormal. I was told that I had human papillomavirus (HPV) and if left untreated it could turn into cervical cancer.

There was a definite severity invoked by the word *cancer*. Even just the possibility of it scared me. Being young and fearful, I listened to my doctor's advice and had a series of colposcopies and several LEEP[i] procedures, where parts of my cervix were removed for biopsy.

I recall the first time I had a scheduled procedure. Shortly before it was about to begin, I called to cancel the appointment. I was afraid. Ryan convinced me that I should go. My health was important—I think he felt the lingering fear of the C-word too. I called back and told the woman on the phone that things had changed and I was going to come in.

I went in alone with a nervous sickness inside of me. The nurse knew that I had called to cancel, and given the look on my face could

i   Loop electrosurgical excision procedure (LEEP) uses a wire loop heated by electric current to remove cells and tissue as part of the diagnosis and treatment for abnormal or cancerous conditions in a woman's lower genital tract tell that I was nervous. When she asked about it I burst into tears. I was alone and frightened and pretty cold in the sterile room. That lovely nurse handed me a tissue for my tears then held my hand during the entire procedure.

I had to follow up with my gynecologist a couple of months later and found out that the abnormality still existed. This was the start of a three-year journey of procedures and follow-up pap smears. The procedures were very painful, like having a needle stuck in my vagina for days. It hurt to pee. I cramped up horribly. I dreaded the calls from the doctor's office that relayed my test results, which continued to show abnormalities in my cervical cells.

The painful procedures became a part of my life. I always went to them alone.

Looking back, I realize that I was embarrassed of what was going on with me. HPV is a sexually transmitted disease and the sound of that made me feel dirty, as if part of the physical pain I had to endure with each procedure was my fault. In reality, I was not the only one with this condition. According to the Centers of Disease Control (CDC) HPV is the most common sexually transmitted infection. It is so common that nearly all sexuality active women will get it at some point in their lives. There are about 14 million people who are newly infected each year.[1]

I couldn't help but feel the shame anyway.

I was always incredibly nervous with each procedure, sitting in the paper gown, alone in the sterile white room. My eyes couldn't help but fall on the tools next to me, all prepared to cause pain to my insides. My gynecologist always picked at the same spot – an area to the right. I bit the inside of my lip and held my breath with hope that it would be over soon.

In between these painful procedures, I started to experience abnormal bleeding during my monthly cycle. This prompted more visits to my gynecologist. I had the routine down. Go pee in a cup, get on the white gown, wait, anticipate, and try not to cry. My gynecologist told me that this bleeding was in fact normal and probably just from my cervix healing.

My mind didn't take this suggestion as truth. My intuition knew better. Something was wrong.

That gynecologist ended up retiring from practice—even though she appeared to be very young—and left me with an associate of hers and a stack of papers that marked the long history of procedures I had endured. I was 24 years old and well aware of just how messed up my insides were. All the picking and probing made this evident. The pain continued past those times in the white sterile room. With it came memories of this physical and emotional trauma.

Instead of remaining with the associate of the retiring gynecologist, I changed to a new gynecologist at a different practice. She did a pap smear and lo and behold, it was clear. These tests remained clear for subsequent checkups, a huge relief. It would be another five years before another doctor would tell me that abnormal pap smears were actually quite common for women in their early to mid-twenties, and that most of the time the immune system was able to clean up those issues without treatment.

It was a statement that made me believe the long, painful years of procedures had never been necessary and likely caused more harm than good. If left alone, my body could have cleared the abnormalities all on its own.

A Question of Faith

Ryan remained by my side. Eventually. With time. From friends to something more. And after five years of many ups and downs, he proposed to me with a song he wrote. He sang it while playing his acoustic guitar then presented me with a beautiful ring that had a yellow sapphire center. That yellow jump-started the color scheme for our wedding six months later.

It was a timeframe that turned out to be incredibly stressful. I didn't realize all the details involved in planning a wedding—all the decisions! When things got down to the wire, I literally turned into a crazy woman. One of the biggest underlying stressors in the process came from a lingering question: in what faith were we going to be married? My parents assumed we were going to get married in the faith I was raised in. A faith that my father dedicated his life to.

I really struggled with this. The inner child in me wanted to please my parents, but my heart was pulling me in the opposite direction. I didn't connect with this chosen faith.

I believe that faith is a very personal choice. Many are raised a certain way and this is who they remain. It is more difficult when an inner resistance conflicts with outer family beliefs. I could have just gone along with it and gotten married the way my parents wanted me to. But instead, I followed the pull in my heart.

God would most definitely be present at our wedding, but not in a traditional, religious setting. He would be there as the wind in the trees and the sunlight reflecting in the pond outside a cute little chapel that faced the magnificent, ancient Red Rocks in Colorado.

The wedding turned out beautiful. Yellow daisies and the simplicity of white surrounded two souls, best friends, joining together as one. Our theme was music. Our invitations were rock concert tickets. We even rocked out on our plastic rock band instruments following our first dance. Epic.

Unfortunately, my decision to not follow a traditional religious wedding left some discontentment with my parents. It drove a deep wedge between us, a pain I tried to swallow, but it lay like a brick in my chest for months to come. I felt like a disappointment to them. Prior to the wedding, my father and I had engaged in a very heated conversation. I tried to get him to understand that I did not connect with his chosen faith and did not feel right about standing in front of everyone pretending to be something I was not.

"What was I then?" he asked.

What was I? Did faith define me? Did it define him? If that was the case, it turned out I didn't have a name for what I was. Did I need a name?

I believe these questions were asked of me at the most opportune moment of my life, preceding a tremendous shift in my life's direction and beliefs about myself.

Who am I?

ROAD
TO
DIAGNOSIS

"Numbing the pain for a while will make it worse when you finally feel it."

~ J.K. Rowling, Harry Potter and the Goblet of Fire

A NEW CHAPTER OF PAIN

During the time when I had been without a doctor, my prescription for birth control ran out and I made the decision not to continue with it. I was tired of the added hormones and wanted to see what life would be like without them. But when I got off of the pill, the pain reawakened in a very, very real way.

My period pain exploded, leaving me shivering in a ball of nausea, diarrhea, and contractions from my uterus that I believe competed with labor pains. This throb persisted for the entire first day of my period, sending pain like shards of glass to the nerves throughout my body.

The new gynecologist reviewed my medical history then listened to me recount the abnormalities I was experiencing and the constant ache on my ride side, the area I was picked at for years. This ache got worse mid-cycle and right before my period. I also described just how bad my periods were.

She scheduled me for an ultrasound, which revealed a cyst on my ovary. She explained that this was likely the cause of my pain. She suggested monitoring it to make sure that it went away on its own. In a couple of weeks the cyst was gone, but the pain on my right side persisted.

After several months of not taking birth control, my periods continued to get progressively worse. I mentioned this to my gynecologist on several occasions and the answer was always the same: take ibuprofen and load up on it prior to your period.

Oh and, "You're sure you don't want to get back on the pill?"

I declined, though as the pain with my periods progressed, I did consider it. However, in the end, I decided to tough it out. I continued to take over the counter pain medication (NSAIDs) on a daily basis, multiple times a day. But the pain just got worse. There were times during my period where I curled into a ball and just moaned.

Nothing touched the pain. I was rendered useless with the start of my period each month and missed work often.

I told myself I could deal with the pain. It was only a few days out of the month. It made me stronger, I reminded myself. Eventually, the pain continued past my periods. It became a daily occurrence, a consistent hurt on my right side that transcended to my hips, lower back, and down to my feet. I was exhausted all the time.

Something definitely wasn't right.

During this same time, I was having spasms of pain that caused my back to go out. I couldn't walk or really move without prompting violent spasms. An MRI showed two herniated discs in my lower back (L4, L5). These bulging discs were hitting on my sciatic nerve.

The doctors told me that I needed surgery, but my gut told me *no*. I didn't want to put pieces of my very delicate nervous system in the hands of a surgeon who could be having an off day. One slip of the wrist and things could get a whole lot worse for me. Unfortunately, surgery or not, things did get a lot worse. My life became consumed by chronic pain, which was exhausting. It became a struggle to wake up each day. It was difficult to concentrate or carry through with anything.

The pain was accompanied by plagues of suffocating depression. I just wanted to crawl into bed and pull the covers over my head, which I did often—too often. My life became a revolving door of emotional highs and lows. The depression was met with sister emotions: anger and resentment. *Why me?* I hated my weak body. I hated that it kept me from living my life to its full potential.

I tried to numb the pain with painkillers. This did the trick for a short period of time until the high wore off and I awoke with the same pain, only worse from the hangover of opiate withdrawal.

Emotional outbursts escalated with Ryan. Screaming matches were met with an exchange of ugly words. At times I felt disassociated from myself, watching a very angry woman that couldn't be me—could it?

Suicidal thoughts surfaced again. I had daydreams about how I would do it. I wondered if anyone would miss me when I was gone. I wondered what they would say at my funeral. I recall several instances of pure emotional turmoil sitting on top of the toilet seat, where all I could look at was the gleam of the razor blade on the edge of the tub. The desire to cut out the emotional pain never left me. I wanted to see it drip out of me.

I think the emotional pain associated with the hormonal imbalances I was experiencing were comparable, if not worse, to the physical pain. I was out of control and hated that feeling more than anything.

I also felt like nobody understood. It was difficult to relay the experience of chronic pain to others who had not experienced it. I tried to defend my actions as a result of something else taking control.

ENDO WHAT...?

I missed yet another day of work at the start of my period and suffered through the next day in my cubicle with my heating pad pressed firmly to my pelvic area. On that day a co-worker suggested a source of my suffering. She gave a name to the monster ripping apart my insides.

She called it endometriosis.

She said that her friend had been struggling with it for a very long time. She had similar, agonizing periods and pain accompanied her pretty much all the time. Her friend also struggled with infertility.

It felt good for someone to take notice of what I was going through and it was good to have an inkling of reasoning behind the pain I was having. I had never heard of endometriosis, so I took to Google and started doing some research on this disease. It was disheartening. Endometriosis was a chronic condition with no cure. Basically, it was where stray cells from the lining of the uterus—the endome-trium— ended up on the outside of the uterus, attaching to other organs, especially in the pelvic region.

These cells acted like they were still part of the uterus, so they continued to thicken with each menstrual cycle and during men-struation they tried to shed. But because no other area of the body is equipped for that kind of shedding in the way the uterus is, these areas would instead become inflamed and scar.

I spent time in support groups reading posts from other women with endometriosis. I could relate so much to their words. Their questions and comments about digestive issues were right in line with mine. Their stories of pain—just like mine. I finally felt a drop of hope, thinking that at least there might be an answer to my symptoms.

How had I never heard of endometriosis? Why had my doctors never mentioned this?

My symptoms persisted. The sharp pain on my right side was ever-present and became worse mid-cycle, right up until my period. I bled after sex, when sex actually happened. As time passed that had become a rarity; it just hurt too much to even try. I felt guilty that I wasn't able to be the sexual type of woman we both yearned for me to be.

Every time I made love with Ryan, I suffered during and after-wards. An act that was supposed to be so intimate and enjoyable became a sore, stressful encounter. I could see his fear each time we attempted to make love, and I forced myself not to flinch, biting the inside of my lip. When the sex was over and followed by blood, it became all that more concerning. Something was definitely wrong.

I made another appointment with my gynecologist to discuss my concerns. She suggested scheduling another ultrasound to see what was going on. Anxious and eager for an answer I scheduled it as soon as I could, I needed a name for the pain I was experiencing. I was pretty sure I had endometriosis but I wanted to hear it from the lips of a medical professional, for my own sanity. The only appointment available was on my 29th birthday, but I scheduled it anyway.

THE LEADING CAUSE OF INFERTILITY

I came in on my lunch hour from work and anxiously waited for my name to be called. Pregnant women surrounded me, big bellies to my left and right and as the time droned on they continued to file in.

The most bothersome find in my research was fact that endometriosis was the leading cause of infertility, representing some 30–40 percent of infertile cases.[2] The pain I'd experienced in my lady parts for much of my life had always created a fear in the back of my mind that I wouldn't be able to have kids, but to have that actually confirmed would be devastating.

While Ryan and I weren't necessarily trying to get pregnant at the time, I'd been off of birth control for three years and we weren't using any other form of protection. We both assumed that getting pregnant was a possibility. It just hadn't happened yet.

With the potential of endometriosis in my body, threatening to spread and damage my reproductive organs, my focus easily shifted towards the fact that pregnancy may not be a possibility after all. What if I was unable to give Ryan the child he had always dreamed about? What was I worth then? Would he still love me? Who wants a woman who's unable to bear a child, that which the female body is designed to do? Sitting in that cramped waiting room, I started to feel sick to my stomach.

Eventually my name was called. I moved to the examination room, undressed, and waited some more. My eyes scanned over the different stages of pregnancy on a chart near the bed, then shifted to a bulletin board overflowing with images of smiling mothers and their beautiful babies. My stomach twisted some more. The ultrasound technician arrived and took a look inside of me. I tried not to flinch as the wand moved through my sore and sensitive pelvic region. I distracted myself by looking at the black and white distorted shapes on the screen, trying to figure out what she was seeing.

She clicked her mouse around and highlighted different areas. She told me she didn't see anything indicating endometriosis but that ultrasounds did not usually detect it. She suggested I chat with the doctor before heading off. That meant I had to return to the waiting room.

It seemed like the pregnant bellies had multiplied. I found a seat and waited. I tried to avoid the scene around me. I felt like I stuck out like a sore thumb. I was the only non-pregnant woman in the room. My emotions continued to roll in waves and threatened to pour from my tear ducts.

I spent the majority of my 29th birthday in that doctor's office waiting on a diagnosis that could significantly alter the remaining part of my life. Would I ever be a mom? Was this the start to a trend in my life? What if I never got answers? What if I never got pregnant? Did the pregnant ladies around me truly understand the miracle they'd been blessed with, to house a new life, to birth someone who shared a piece of their soul?

These emotions built up inside of me as I waited, alone.

ALL SIGNS POINT TO ENDOMETRIOSIS

Eventually my name was called and I went back to consult with my gynecologist. I laid out my symptoms for her again: the constant ache in my pelvic region, my ovaries, hips, lower back. I was bleeding at different parts of my cycle, spotting five days prior to the start of my period, and spotting after sex. Sex was painful and my period pain was off the charts.

She nodded her head, listening. I paused and waited for the diagnosis I sought after spending hours researching and being a fly on the wall in endometriosis support groups. But she did not suggest it. I did.

"I think I have endometriosis," I said. My voice wavered.

She nodded some more and agreed it was a possibility, but the only way to know for sure was to have a laparoscopic surgical procedure where the doctor went in and looked around the pelvic region. If endometriosis was found, it was removed.

"You're sure you don't want to get back on the pill?" she asked.

I shook my head. "Are there other options available if it is endometriosis?"

She told me about Lupron, a drug that essentially kicked the body into menopause. Luckily, I knew of this drug after spending time in support groups. I knew it was a terrible drug that had devastating, long-term side effects.

"If this is endometriosis, then it could affect my fertility, right?" I already knew the answer to the question but I asked it anyways, because I couldn't get the thought out of my head: my insides were broken.

"Yes," she said.

My pent up emotions hit a breaking point and the tears I'd been fighting shook out in fat droplets of pain that splattered on the linoleum floor. My breath shook with a wave of grief, pure frustration, and animosity for the pain in my body, for the robbing of potential new life from the very center of me.

After witnessing my breakdown, she offered me a prescription for anti-depressants. I declined. Instead, I left with a card for a psychotherapist who dealt with chronic pain, as well as a slim bit of hope that the ravaging pain would someday cease. I spent the rest of my 29th birthday in tears, starting with intermittent rounds of sobbing in my cubicle at work and going well into the night, where my sadness was drowned in beers and comfort food.

The days that followed were some of my worst on record. I had violent mood swings and fell into weeks of depression. I did not want to leave the confines of my bed. I hated my body and even more so the pain it brought. I was exhausted.

Tension between Ryan and I intensified. We were in the beginning years of our marriage. Most couples were likely much more intimate than we were. I had lost the desire. My libido was slim to none and the pain associated with sex just wasn't worth it.

Still, I waited four months before finally opting to have the surgery. While I was pretty sure that I had endometriosis, I needed the diagnosis to confirm it. I needed to know, beyond a shadow of a doubt—both for myself and for those around me who didn't understand the depths of my chronic pain.

I looked fine on the outside. Meanwhile, my insides were on fire.

CUTTING IN TO BE SURE

On April 26, 2011, I had laparoscopic surgery. I was 13 days into my cycle. I had to do bowel prep and struggled over 24 hours only consuming liquids. I haven't been able to enjoy vegetable broth the same since.

The surgery was the week following Easter. Ryan and I were gifted an Easter basket loaded full of sweet goodies. By the end of my day of fasting, I could smell the sugar protruding from that basket and felt a little crazy coming on. Especially when I saw him devouring pieces from it.

I somehow made it through without any food and rode in my famished state to the hospital with Ryan and my mother-in-law by my side. This was my first surgery where I had to go completely under and a part of me was uneasy. My intuition told me that something was wrong with the whole process; that I had to undergo a surgical procedure to have proof of a disease inside of me, with a doctor I hoped that I could trust going in with a laser and removing what he found out of place.

I gulped as I signed the release stating the risks involved with the surgery, including death. A possibility. Was this all worth it?

Filled with fear, famine, and an inner frustration my stomach twisted when I kissed Ryan goodbye and was wheeled in a hospital bed down a long corridor of white walls and buzzing fluorescent lights. I had a short look around the operating room at the faces ready to assist in cutting me open to have a look inside. They had the opportunity to see what the pain looked like.

One of the nurses had a pair of red plastic devil horns on her head. I kid you not. This was the last image I had before I went under. I woke up in the recovery area and immediately felt a stabbing in my insides. I'm not sure I had much of a voice to cry out, but one of the nurses must have noticed my painful awakening. I gratefully accepted more pain medication, which really only dulled this new, horrible pain in my center and made me super nauseous, which certainly didn't help things.

Ryan and my mother in law greeted me and helped me out of the wheelchair and into the car. On the way home I avoided looking out at the passing scenery. Instead I focused much of my energy levels on not puking all over myself.

I had very little recollection of the doctor's debriefing after my surgery, but I gathered that I did, indeed, have endometriosis. It was on the outside of my uterus and ovaries and in the area around my uterus.

Once I had time to rest and overcome the anesthesia I looked through the packet of images they had taken of the endometrial implants during surgery. They kind of looked like blood blisters. The images served almost as a souvenir from my $10,000 surgery. At least they were proof of all I had been experiencing. This was what the pain looked like.

I finally had a diagnosis. A name for the pain I had suffered with for so many years. But did the name really change anything except to provide certainty on something that intuitively I already knew.

I popped more pain pills and soaked in the high that helped remove my mind from the pain radiating from my center. I looked down at the bandages on each hip and my belly button covering the incision sites. True warrior scars.

WHAT ABOUT MY FERTILITY?

I was anxious to meet again with the surgeon to see what his thoughts were after surgery, especially in regards to my fertility. While I was under, they had done a test to see if there were any blockages in my tubes, but that came back fine. He didn't see anything wrong physically that should prevent me from getting pregnant, and explained that he had removed all the endometriosis he could find.

Still, simply having endometriosis would be a negative impact on my fertility. The doctor told me that the longer I waited, the harder it would likely be to get pregnant. He suggested either getting back on birth control or trying to conceive as soon as possible.

I squeezed Ryan's hand. While we'd talked about wanting kids, I didn't feel right confirming this big life decision in my paper gown, still sore from being cut open, gassed up and sewn back together. I wasn't exactly in a sexy kind of mind. But we figured it couldn't hurt to get checked out further for fertility factors. Everything from those tests came back good. There was little reason to believe we shouldn't be able to get pregnant—at least on paper.

To ensure that those chances remained solid, we were even invited by my doctor to participate in a fertility drug study where I would essentially be a guinea pig for different fertility drugs. This didn't feel right to either of us; we were going to give it a good old-fashioned try on our own first.

WHAT NOW?

After having a concrete diagnosis, I had to figure out what I was going to do next. Endometriosis was devastating because in many ways it felt like it was out of my control. From the dawn of my diagnosis I heard:

- "There is no cure for endometriosis."
- "It will only get worse."
- "It will negatively affect your fertility."
- "You may never get pregnant."

The doctor's authority conditioned me to believe that endometriosis was incurable and chronic. When labeled this way, my mind was subconsciously programmed with negative beliefs.

All of these realities felt very much out of my control, which only served to stress and depress me. I couldn't imagine carrying on forever with chronic pain. That possibility left me with a sense of hopelessness and sadness. The doctors offered me few options: birth control pills; Lupron, which limits estrogen production; or to get pregnant as soon as possible.

My intuition whispered that drugs were not the way to conquer it. I'd already spent a third of my young life on artificial hormones. I didn't want to go back down that path. The latter option of pregnancy *was* an option. However, I understood that before I was going to get pregnant, I would need to somehow take care of this newly named inner monster, especially considering sex was still a very painful endeavor.

There had to be another way.

To find an alternate path to managing this newly named disease, which threatened a life of never-ending pain, I went back to researching.

LESSON ONE:
FOOD
IS THE
FOUNDATION

" Let food be thy medicine,
and medicine be thy food."

~Hippocrates

THE IMPACT OF FOOD

This time I shifted my research towards natural methods of treating endometriosis. What I found were stories of other women with the condition who were able to manage their pain through dietary changes. My world opened up when I discovered the crucial link between the pain and inflammation in my body and the food that I was eating.

Prior to this discovery, I didn't cook for myself. Instead, I relied on fast food restaurants to fill my body with French fries, hamburgers, and milk shakes. In turn, my body was in a constant state of inflammation from the food in my standard American diet (SAD).

Throughout the years of bloating, gas, headaches, joint pain, and painful periods, I'd never put two and two together. In reality, the food that I ate was transformed to the cells in my body and made up my blood, tissues, and organs. My cells relied on nutrients to fully function. When my body received low levels of nutrients it caused my cellular processes to fail. Add endometriosis to the mix—inflammatory blood pockets where they shouldn't be—and it's no wonder I was a big bloated mess most of the time.

FOOD AND INFLAMMATION

As I made more discoveries about the impacts of food and inflammatory reactions in my body, I learned about the important balance between anti-inflammatory and inflammatory lipid hormones called prostaglandins (PGs). The endometrium—the tissue that lines the womb—is an important endocrine gland and secretes a family of PGs that are directly responsible for most of the cramps and pain associated with menstruation and endometriosis.

There are two prostaglandins in particular that are problematic: prostaglandin F (PGF), which stimulates strong uterine contractions or cramps, and prostaglandin E (PGE), which triggers excruciating pain.

Large amounts of PGF and PGE are produced by your endometrium. With endometriosis the endometrium is found outside your womb, but these cells still react like they are part of your womb. The endometrium and its straying implants are very responsive to the levels of PGs circulating in your blood.

At the end of your menstrual cycle there is a natural surge of PGF that signals the start of a new menstrual cycle. Learning this helped me to understand why the start of my period was often the most painful part. PGF also increases gut motility leading to irritable bowel syndrome (IBS) and diarrhea. This helped explain why my periods started off with significant bowel movements.

Not all prostaglandins are bad, however. There are three different types:

- Series 1 (linoleic acid)
- Series 2 (arachidonic acid)
- Series 3 (alpha-linolenic acid).

Linoleic acid is derived from vegetable oils including safflower, sunflower, hemp, walnuts, pumpkin seeds, and sesame seeds. Alpha-linolenic acid is derived from fish and linseed oils. Both linoleic acid and alpha-linolenic acid are anti-inflammatory. Arachidonic acid is inflammatory and comes primarily from dairy foods and meat.

I learned that these three different types of prostaglandins needed to be kept in balance. If too much of the wrong type of PG is produced by our tissues, then internal inflammation and pain occurs. An imbalance causes pre-menstrual syndrome (PMS) and endometriosis pain.

The balance of these prostaglandins is largely dependent on the quality of fats and oils that we consume. Needless to say, the oils and low quality meat from the fast food that I was eating were full of bad prostaglandins. If I was going to be able to get the pain under control, this habit needed to change.

MY GOOD FRIEND SUGAR

In addition to my frequent fast food stops, I used to have stashes of sweets in my dresser drawers. My favorite was a sweet snack cake that came in vanilla and chocolate, topped with a sweet, ribbed frosting. I would finish off a box of twelve in a couple of days. I tried to keep this habit out of sight, but I was unable to hide it from Ryan. He spotted the empty treat boxes and shook his head.

"You're going to get fat if you keep eating those like that," he teased.

That word *fat* rang through my mind. While this didn't help me to control the sugar binges, it did prompt me to start working out. I spent a lot of time doing cardio and attempting the different weight machine contraptions at the gym. I ran and I ran, but the weight really didn't shift. So I ran some more.

I felt guilty each time I indulged on the sweet stuff but didn't stop. I just did a better job of hiding it and I made sure to run some more. I was working out all the time thinking that was the way to lose weight without taking into consideration what I was eating.

The high that came from my sugar binges was super addictive. With one taste of it, I only wanted more and more. Sugar invoked an emotional connection within me, sparking its use during times of stress for comfort. This is because sugar releases endorphins or feel-good hormones in our bodies, a reaction that leads to further consumption once the high crashes.

The human body is naturally inclined to crave sugar for survival. The brain is wired to want it. The problem was, I was taking in way too much of it. This wrecked havoc on my insulin levels.

SUGAR AND INSULIN RESISTANCE

I'd never really considered insulin, or honestly, even knew what it was. Turns out it's a pretty big deal. Insulin is a hormone produced by your pancreas. It acts as a messenger between your cells. With the help of insulin, cells throughout your body absorb glucose and use it for energy.

Glucose is a form of sugar that enters your bloodstream after eating carbohydrates and starches. Insulin helps muscle, fat, and liver cells absorb glucose from your bloodstream, thereby lowering blood glucose levels. Your pancreas has to produce insulin in order to maintain normal blood sugar levels. If it has to do this too much then issues arise. Rapid changes in blood sugar levels can stimulate cravings and increases the likelihood of systemic inflammation.

I ate way too many high-glycemic foods including white bread, cookies, cakes, bagels, etc. This resulted in glycemic stress and inflammation of my blood vessels. Over time, the blood vessel lining thickens, making it more and more difficult for the insulin to get out and into our cells, signaling the production of inflammatory chemicals.

Glycemic stress and inflammation eventually leads to insulin resistance. With this condition our bodies produce insulin but do not use it effectively. So glucose builds up in our blood instead of being absorbed by our cells.

When insulin levels are off then our bodies have a hard time losing weight because when your cells are constantly producing more insulin, they are not turning insulin into needed nutrients and energy. Your cells become starved and your body holds on to what it can. This helped explain why I was not losing weight in between my sugar binging episodes.

It should be noted that having this extra weight on my body was not a good thing for endometriosis as excess estrogen in my body—

the fuel for endometriosis—gathered in my fat cells.

Insulin also affects ovarian function. Your ovaries are very sensitive to insulin, as it makes your ovary produce testosterone. Too much insulin can cause too many ovarian follicles to be stimulated. This can lead to ovarian cysts. Something I was definitely prone to.

Insulin resistance has ties to polycystic ovary syndrome (PCOS), as high insulin triggers high levels of the hormones testosterone and LH, which leads to anovulation, where your ovaries fail to produce a viable egg. Excess insulin, therefore, can affect pregnancy, as it prevents ovulation.

According to Dr. Christiane Northrup in her book, *Women's Bodies, Women's Wisdom*, signs of insulin abuse include:[3]

- carbohydrate cravings and uncontrollable hunger;
- emotional eating;
- night time eating;
- resistance to weight loss; and
- fatigue and shakiness after eating.

Signs of impending insulin resistance also include low HDL cholesterol, increased triglycerides, heartburn, hypoglycemia, and insomnia.

Do you relate to these symptoms as much as I did?

SUGAR AND THE IMMUNE SYSTEM

I learned that sugar also suppresses our immune system and upsets mineral relationships in our bodies. It interferes with our bodies' ability to absorb calcium and magnesium, both of which aide in the reduction of cramps. Sugar also increases reactive oxygen species (ROS), thus causing damage to our cells and tissues.

Sugar reduces your body's ability to defend itself from infection as it feeds organisms like the candida fungus, which has been linked to endometriosis. Candida leaves behind traces of estrogen in your body, which feeds endometriosis.

The break out of sugar-free products is not any better. Many of these products contain aspartame, a poison linked to plenty of neurological issues including headaches, migraines, dizziness, nausea, numbness, muscle spasms, weight gain, rashes, depression, fatigue, joint pain, and on and on.

Aspartame is made up of three ingredients: aspartic acid, phenylalanine, and methanol. It was developed in a lab, not in Mother Nature. The high experienced from aspartame is the party in your brain as its cells die.

With this information under my belt, I understood that I needed to break up with sugar if I was ever going to stop the inflammation in my body.

Finding a New Way of Eating

Desperate for relief from the pain, I decided to cut out a number of these inflammatory foods. In a whim one day at lunch with Ryan, I pushed the food aside. I set an intention then and there that I was going to eat differently.

Problem was, inflammatory foods made up my diet and I didn't really know how to cook. I didn't know what to eat. I started pretty simple: beans and rice. Those two staples made up pretty much all my meals at first, before I slowly started adding in more vegetables.

Eventually I figured it out. This was a huge change for me, but I stuck with it.

I found something that gave me a sense of control over this disease, and it didn't come in a pill bottle.

I was quite rigid with my dietary restrictions at first:

Can't eat that.

Nope.

No thank you.

I felt like an outcast, the one not eating or eating very little at social events. Awkward conversations always followed my food refusal. I quickly developed an elevator speech as to why I was not eating the provided food. In short, I explained how these foods didn't make me feel good and how I would face consequences later if I did eat them. Usually that was enough. With the commonality of food allergies these days, most people understood.

While these food changes drew attention to me, it was worth it because I really felt better. And in turn, those pounds I'd been running and running to lose just melted off. People noticed that as well.

Eventually I cut out alcohol because it just plain made me feel horrible. Then I was the sober girl who didn't eat anything.

I couldn't help but feel like the weird one. I always struggled with the notion of fitting in and these change made this more difficult. In spite of my social status, I stayed disciplined. But discipline is like a muscle. It takes training. And it is always being tested. Eventually, my discipline muscle wore out and the foods I was working to avoid made their way back in. This was not a big surprise considering my environment was inundated with processed, inflammatory foods.

Everywhere I went I came across unhealthy foods.

After a while I tested the water and tried introducing these inflammatory foods back into my diet. And the pain returned, in my hips, my joints. And my body responded; I was bloated, gassy, tired, had headaches, my sinuses were clogged, and my skin broke out. Only when I started to feel better did I realize just how bad I had been feeling. I'd known no different before.

EATING TO HEAL ENDOMETRIOSIS

There were times on my journey when I stressed out about the impacts of every little thing I was eating. I wondered sometimes if my own fears about what to eat did more harm than good. If you have done your own research you already know how many nutritional theories contradict each other and how the process of eating for healing can become quite confusing and frustrating.

It took me a while to figure out that what I needed to do was reconnect with the signals and symptoms my body was giving me. An easy way to track how your food is making you feel is with a journal. Simply jot down what you eat every day and how you feel afterwards. Take a moment and scan over your body. Did the food you ate have an impact on how you feel? A food journal is also helpful for tracking emotional eating patterns that could be playing a role in food choices.

The easiest way to see if a food is the causative factor behind pain in your body or digestive troubles is to eliminate it from your diet for three to four weeks then reintroduce the food back in and see how you feel afterwards.

Everyone's body is different. What may be good for one could be like poison to another. It takes a connection with your body to figure out how you feel when you add in and subtract foods. Your body truly knows best. Trust your gut on this one.

That being said, I have provided suggested food guidelines below and some reasoning as to why we should add and avoid certain things. This list should help you get started on feeling better with endometriosis.

The addition and elimination of ingredients is a lifestyle change, but if I can do it, you can do it!

Foods to Add

Omega-3 Oils. Anti-inflammatory; helps balance out bad prostaglandins.

Found in oily fish, walnuts, pumpkin seeds, dark green leafy vegetables, Omega-3 fortified eggs, hemp seeds. To ensure that I am getting a good balance of good prostaglandins every day, I also supplement with a high dose of quality fish oil tablets.

Fiber. Helps move out bad estrogens through the digestive tract, which fuel endometriosis. The best source of easy to digest fiber is in fruits and vegetables.

Full color spectrum of fruits and vegetables. Fruits and vegetables are full of such wonderful nutrition to help heal our bodies. The fresher the better and organic is the best choice.

Cruciferous vegetables. Full of healing vitamins such as zinc, A, B, C, D, and E. More importantly, cruciferous vegetables contain indole-3-carbinol (I3C) that participates in the metabolism of bad estrogens. Examples include broccoli, cauliflower, cabbage, kale, bok choi, and Brussels sprouts

Note: Cruciferous vegetables contain goitrogens that can cause an enlargement of your thyroid gland. In addition, they can act like an anti-thyroid drug, slowing down your thyroid ultimately causing hypothyroidism. To avoid this effect, cruciferous vegetables should be consumed lightly cooked or steamed.

Good fats. Your sex hormones are synthesized from cholesterol in your ovaries and your adrenal glands. Your body also uses cholesterol to make bile in your liver so it's very important to include healthy fat sources in avocados, nuts, seeds, and if desired, hormone-free, antibiotic-free, grass-fed animal sources.

Cold pressed olive oil is another good choice, though it should only be consumed raw. When cooked, many oils turn rancid and cause free radicals to roam through your body, causing further inflammation. The best oils to cook with are coconut oil, grape seed oil, or avocado oil as they have a higher smoke point before going rancid.

Foods with a lower glycemic load. Monitoring the glycemic load of different foods helps keep blood sugar levels balanced and increase a hormone that regulates the metabolism of fat and sugar. Studies suggest that there is a correlation between glycemic load and systemic inflammation.[4] Foods with a glycemic load of 10 or less is good. Most fruits and vegetables have a lower glycemic load.

Cinnamon. Cinnamon assists with heavy menstrual bleeding and assists with circulation. It also contains a natural compound called cinnamaldehyde that naturally increases the sex hormone progesterone, which most women with endometriosis are lacking in.

Apple cider vinegar (ACV). ACV has a myriad of benefits for healing endometriosis. It is high in acetic acid, which helps your body absorb important minerals from the food you eat. It also binds to toxins so that they are more efficiently eliminated from your body. In addition, ACV helps break up mucus in your body and helps to cleanse your lymph nodes, break up gallstones in your gallbladder, and detoxifies your liver. It normalizes blood sugar levels and has an alkalinizing effect on your body. Taking a tablespoon in water ten minutes or so before eating helps to aide in your digestive process.

Filtered water. Dehydration adds to the aches and pains of endometriosis. Water helps move out toxins and waste from your body.

FOODS TO AVOID/ELIMINATE

Wheat, barley, rye. These grains contain a high amount of phytic acid, which prevents the absorption of vitamins and minerals. It also contains gluten, which causes inflammation and contributes to leaky gut.

Refined carbohydrates and sugar. This includes white flours and sugars and makes up most processed pastas, cakes, cookies, and other treats. These foods have a higher glycemic load and cause inflammation in your body.

Note: To keep sugar cravings at bay, I found it helpful to start the day with protein and fat, rather than just carbohydrates. This helped level out blood sugar levels for the day and kept my body from experiencing a late afternoon crash.

Dairy. Stimulates bad prostaglandins causing inflammation and pain. Much of the dairy produced these days contains hormones and other unwanted additives that are no good for endometriosis.

Hydrogenated oils. These bad oils also stimulate bad prostaglandins and free radicals that cause damage to your body causing inflammation and pain.

Soy. Soy is very hard to digest and much of the non-organic soy in the United States is genetically modified, which makes it even harder for the body to process. Soy contains a large amount of phytoestrogens that can aggravate endometriosis, especially if the liver is not healthy, common among women with endometriosis. Small amounts of fermented soy are all right in moderation.

Note: I understand how difficult soy is to avoid completely. I gave up early on totally eliminating the small bits of it that are added to so many things.

Food additives and preservatives. These include anything at the end of the ingredient list that is not natural. If you cannot pronounce it or know what it is, then better to avoid it! Watch out for coloring such as blue 1, red 40, yellow 6, etc. These dyes are horrible for digestion and have been linked to behavioral disorders. Also linked into this category are sulfites, nitrates, etc.

Monosodium glutamate (MSG). MSG is an endocrine disruptor, causing an abnormal hormone release from your thyroid, adrenals, and ovaries. MSG has been shown to cause your ovaries to shrink, leading to reproductive issues. Larger doses of it can lower thyroid levels. I've found that MSG is usually added to chicken products. Most fast food companies use it as a flavor enhancer for their chicken and it is also found in most packaged chicken products such as chicken broth.

MSG can also appear as:

- autolyzed yeast extract

- glutamate
- monopotassium glutamate
- textured protein
- yeast nutrient
- calcium caseinate
- glutamic acid
- yeast extract
- hydrolyzed vegetable protein
- hydrolyzed protein
- gelatin
- sodium caseinate
- yeast food
- natural flavoring
- spices

Sugary drinks and alcohol. Sugar increases inflammation as does alcohol. Alcohol wears on your liver and is said to increase estrogen levels.

Citrus fruits. The elimination of citrus fruits is an individual choice. Citrus can irritate your stomach and can upset the way in which estrogen is excreted by your body. However, many citrus fruits, including limes and lemons are beneficial for your liver and kidneys. Pay attention to how you feel afterwards to see if you are sensitive. Many women with endometriosis also suffer from a sister disease called interstitial cystitis, or painful bladder syndrome. If you experience pain in your bladder then it may be helpful to avoid citrus foods.

Note: If a food is upsetting digestion then it is causing an immune system response and should be avoided.

BUY ORGANIC WHEN POSSIBLE

To avoid the negative consequences from many of the poisons and hormone altering chemicals sprayed on our foods, it is best to buy everything possible organic. If this is not possible, then at least stay away from the Environmental Working Group's Dirty Dozen and lean towards produce in the Clean 15.

The Environmental Working Group is a nonprofit organization in support of individual health. They tested the produce after it was washed to see how much residue remained from pesticides sprayed on the produce. The dirty dozen had the highest pesticide load and the clean 15 had the lowest pesticide load. The following foods were on the 2014 results.

The dirty dozen:

> apples
> strawberries
> grapes
> celery
> peaches
> spinach
> sweet bell peppers
> nectarines
> cucumbers
> cherry tomatoes
> snap peas
> potatoes

The clean 15:

> avocados
> sweet corn
> pineapples
> cabbage
> sweet peas (frozen)
> onions

asparagus

mangoes

papayas

kiwi

eggplant

grapefruit

cantaloupe (domestic)

cauliflower

sweet potatoes

For more information visit www.ewg.org

AVOID GENETICALLY MODIFIED FOODS (GMOs)

In 1996 genetically modified organisms (GMOs) were introduced to the food supply. GMOs are seeds that have been genetically engineered to resist pests and herbicides. Essentially the bugs that try to eat these GMO crops get blown up from the inside. This made me wonder what these GMO foods did to the inside of my gut!

Proponents of GMOs claim that they are necessary to feed the world. The biggest player in the GMO game is a chemical company called Monsanto, which asserts that there are no dangers associated with consuming GMOs, even though lab studies continue to prove otherwise.

The consumption of GMOs can cause overly negative effects on the health of your immune system primarily because of their impact in your digestive tract.[5] Take a look around and it's hard not to notice the exponential rise in food allergies since GMOs hit the market.

GMOs have also been linked to fertility issues, as those who consume them on a regular basis have a harder time getting and staying pregnant. In one European study, rats that were fed GMO food gave birth to pups that died within weeks of birth[6].

The foods most likely to be GMO in the United States include:

- alfalfa
- corn (canola)
- cotton (cottonseed oils)
- soy
- papayas
- zucchini
- yellow summer squash

EMOTIONAL EATING PATTERNS

I learned pain was eminent with the wrong food choices. However, plenty of times I caved to instant gratification over pain later. When I fell off the wagon, I succumbed to feelings of guilt mixed with anger for my body that no longer accepted junk food without a scream.

Other times, in a weird way, I think I wanted to feel the pain. This was during times of emotional distress where my inner emotional pain was so deep that those forbidden foods seemed more appealing because their end result was physical discomfort. Perhaps this was my way of making the emotional pain more physical, more real, more apparent; or perhaps sometimes I hurt emotionally in ways that I felt should hurt in a physical sense.

Later, I recognized that my patterns of binging on sugar were an attempt to fill myself up in an emotional sense. Every time the stress flared, sugar wasn't too far behind. Every time I felt broken, sad, or alone sugar was there to fill me up. I was trying to fill myself up with the sweetness.

Something deeper was missing from my life.

FOOD FOR THE SOUL

In her book, *Women, Food, and God*, emotional eating expert Geneen Roth helped me to discover an important connection between the food that I was eating and the value that I put on my body. This was in greater connection with my soul and even greater connection to a higher power. Her suggestions helped me stop prior to eating something and reflect: How am I feeling? Am I really hungry for food or am I trying to fill up because of some other emotion, whether it was boredom, stress, anxiety, fatigue, sadness, etc.?

This information helped me put together my stress-sugar connection. With this awareness and the practice of discovery, my recurring binging episodes fell further and farther between. Of greater importance, I recognized that it was necessary for me to work towards a healthy body, as it is the physical home for my soul, which is so much bigger.

With the changes that I made in my diet I started to feel better. The bloating, gas, headaches, joint pain, and cramping that I was accustomed to became a rarity. Once I started to feel better, it motivated me to take further care of myself. The shift to nourishing food in my body has allowed me to heal physically so I am more equipped to face challenges and heal internally, in whole.

LESSON TWO: HEALTHY DIGESTION IS KEY

"All disease begins in the gut."

~ Hippocrates

PINPOINTING THE PATH TO HEALING

While I've laid out the dos and don'ts for eating to heal endometriosis, I understand that these changes are not easy. We live in a day and age when it can be a struggle to eat a different way and to stand up for the health and well being of our bodies.

Many a time I watched as others consumed these foods with little to no side effects. This begged the question: Why? Why did I have to restrict myself from the food all around me when others could eat that way and experience no issues?

I recognized that everyone is different, but I wanted to understand why I was *so* different? Why did these foods aggravate me so much? And why, after years of complaining about pain and inflammation in my body, did my gynecologists not suggest food for healing? These questions guided me to further research and a natural pull to alternative ways of healing. I became drawn to teachings from ancient practices such as Chinese medicine and Ayurveda.[ii] I was also drawn to more modern alternative approaches to healing in areas such as integrative and functional medicines.

I found these methods of healing appealing because they looked at the systems in my body as a whole, functioning unit. Endometriosis was not simply confined to my reproductive organs; multiple systems were impacted. Whole healing was necessary. Additionally, the focus that these healing modalities had on balance and appreciation for my unique constitution helped me to understand my body was different because of my physical and emotional make-up.

Most importantly, these teachings helped me pinpoint the center for healing: the digestive tract. According to Ayurveda, digestion is the gateway to our physical, mental, and emotional health. I learned that the food that I needed to eliminate was aggravating this vital system in my body. Each time that I ate out of bounds I was ulti-

ii   Ayurveda is ancient science of curing diseases using natural processes.

mately creating damage to my healing path.

Once I understood just how important of a role food choices played in the digestive tract, I was more motivated to stick with the recommended food choices. I hope that by sharing further knowledge of the digestive process it motivates you too.

ENDOMETRIOSIS AND THE IMMUNE SYSTEM

With endometriosis, cells from the uterus ended up attaching to other places outside the uterus. While there were theories as to why this happened, there was no concrete evidence one way of the other so the cause of endometriosis remains a mystery.

Of all the theories, I personally believe endometriosis is related to my faulty immune system. Whether my immune system caused endometriosis or if the endometriosis damaged my immune system, either way my immune system was failing to do its job. It was supposed to protect my body from danger, but it was weakened along the way and wasn't able to do its job. In theory, since my body was not able to clean up those stray endometrial implants, endometriosis was formed. With this in mind, it seemed to me that the clearest form of action to dissolve endometriosis was to improve the functioning of my immune system.

As mentioned, a key lesson that I learned on my path to healing endometriosis was the importance of healthy digestion. I found out that nearly 80 percent of my immune system is located in the wall of my gut. That was the first line of immune defense in my body and should have excluded toxins, infectious agents, and allergenic material. It's kind of like our inner skin.

IS YOUR GUT LEAKING?

This lining to our intestines is made of cells that are supposed to be connected tightly together. However, a condition called leaky gut destroyed those cells so that large pieces of undigested food, microbes, and toxins got into my body where they were absorbed by my blood stream then detected by my immune system as not belonging. In response, antibodies were released to attack these foreign entities. The more I ate, the more antibodies that were produced until my body developed a chronic inflammatory reaction.

This immune system reaction created symptoms of typical food sensitivities that were a normal part of my life including gas, bloating, constipation, diarrhea, brain fog, fatigue, skin rashes, headaches, joint, and/or muscle pain.

Note: If you have multiple food sensitivities then you likely have leaky gut.

I learned a lot about leaky gut and other factors in the digestive process from a functional doctor named Susan Blum. Functional medicine addresses the underlying causes of disease and approaches healing form a whole body perspective. Dr. Blum describes your intestinal tract as a stream. If there are any breaks or blockages along the way, then the stream is disrupted and issues arise.

In order to heal the delicate gut lining, Dr. Blum recommends removing foods that are causing sensitivities for at least six months, as immune cells have a memory of these foreign invaders and will continue to attack them if not given enough time away from them. The foods that cause the most common food allergies are gluten, dairy, and soy—all items I had eliminated from my diet. When re-introduced them back into my diet, my body reacted.

Once I understood that these foods were causing a damaging immune system response in my body, it made more sense to continue avoiding them. Additional foods that can cause sensitivities include corn and eggs, but I didn't notice as big of a reaction with these so I still eat them in moderation.

Since removing problematic foods from my diet I noticed a significant reduction in pain and a vast improvement in digestive functioning. Some three years later, my sensitivities lessened quite a bit. When these problematic foods slipped back into my diet, the result was not as dramatic as it once had been. But I was still left feeling less than great, so I opted to stay away. My cravings for gluten and dairy have nullified. I don't miss them. I have found that feeling better is worth the sacrifice.

WHAT CAUSES LEAKY GUT?

I am pretty sure that I had leaky gut as I put a lot of things in my body that damaged my intestinal lining and contributed to this condition. These included:
- birth control (for a long period of time)
- lots of doses of antibiotics throughout my life
- pain pills
- over-the-counter NSAIDs

My gut wall was also destroyed by gluten sensitivity and by candida, a yeast that lives in your digestive tract. It can get out of hand if it is overfed with sugar, yeast, and dairy foods. Birth control pills feed candida too and antibiotics are quick to disrupt the balance of good gut flora downstream.

With leaky gut, candida escaped my intestines and set up shop wherever it could find space for growth. The problem with candida is that it has receptor sites, which accept hormones. So if progesterone binds to candida it fails to reach its destination. In addition, candida is said to leave behind traces of estrogen, which only fed endometriosis.

I learned that women with endometriosis are at a higher risk for candida growth, partly due to a disturbance in the microorganisms in our gut. Endometriosis is directly associated with gut inflammation. Some signs that I had candida overgrowth were the frequent infections I experienced including urinary tract infections (UTI) and yeast infections. These annoying, painful issues were popping up every couple of months. Before I knew better, I treated them with antibiotics, which only added to the problem.

Once I learned about candida and its impact on these recurring infections and the negative impacts of antibiotics, I found several natural herbs to help eliminate my candida overgrowth including:

- lemongrass
- clove
- cinnamon
- melaleuca
- pau d'arco

CHEW, CHEW, CHEW

I want to back up for a moment, as a lot happens in your digestive process before the food you eat hits your gut. The digestive process actually starts in your mouth with the act of chewing. Saliva is a key factor in the process as it lubricates the food, making it easier to pass through your esophagus. Saliva also contains enzymes that contribute to your digestive process. By chewing your food you relax the pylorus, a muscle at the end of your stomach. When this muscle is relaxed then food is more readily moved through your digestive tract.

When food I ate was not chewed and large chunks of food went in, incomplete digestion occurred. These chunks of food were more likely to get stuck in my digestive tract lending way to a breeding ground for bad bacteria. When I ate too fast many times I had undigested food in my stools—a signal that my body was not absorbing the nutrients from the food that I was eating.

I really struggled with slowing down when eating. My life was rushed and eating was kind of a chore. My lunches at work were short and my life outside of work was busy. I ate quickly so that I could move on to whatever else I had to do. To help me slow down, I made a point to give full attention to my food. This meant removing the distractions that often accompanied my meals like reading, watching TV, browsing the Internet, working, or even walking while eating. When I was distracted, not enough attention was paid to the act of eating. I just gulped down the food without taking in the true flavor of things.

Distracted eating is said to lead to weight gain. I can see how this would be true because it took my attention away from just how much food I was consuming and my body's signals that it was full. In ways of mindful eating, I made a point to start eating my meals sitting at the kitchen table with no distractions and only focus on my food. When at work, I developed a habit of eating lunch at my desk. Instead, I stepped away and ate my food at a table away from my work environment, undistracted.

By removing distractions and focusing on my food I found re-newed pleasure in the act of eating, of tastes and textures and subtle appreciation that the food was going to nourish my body. This atten-tion also helped me focus on the very important factor in digestion: chewing my food!

IMPACTS OF LOW STOMACH ACID

Once chewed—or unchewed food—enters your mouth it makes its way through the esophagus to your stomach. My research brought light to the vital connection of a properly functioning stomach in the digestive process, which again, affects the correct performance of your immune system.

Dr. Blum taught me the importance of stomach acid. The pH of this acid should be 1.5, which is very acidic in order to kill viruses and bacteria that may be ingested and prevent unwanted infections. Good bacteria are very tolerant of this acid, while unfriendly bacteria and yeast like candida are not. Therefore, it is important to have adequate amounts of stomach acid and a proper pH to keep a balance of good bacteria in your small intestine downstream.

The correct pH is also necessary for the efficient absorption of many vitamins and minerals. Calcium and magnesium are unable to absorb in alkaline pH and the absorption of zinc, a key player in our immune system, is also affected.

Stress, alcohol, H.phylori, aspirin and other medications could all wear away your stomach lining, making it raw and sensitive to the amount of acid that should be in your stomach, a condition known as heartburn. Throughout my life I was definitely no stranger to stress or downing shots of Tequila. I was accustomed to popping pain pills and over-the-counter NSAIDs every day, multiple times a day, depending on my pain levels.

Low stomach acid impairs digestion of proteins especially, which provide the body with amino acids that are needed for the creation of immune cells. In order to have enough of these amino acids the protein needs to digest properly so that it is absorbed in the body. Stomach acid helps activate digestive enzymes so that this happens. Stomach acid is made in special stomach cells called parietal cells. When my stomach was constantly irritated these cells became damaged and produced less acid and less digestive enzymes.

According to Dr. Susan Blum, signs of low stomach acid include:[7]
- bloating/belching immediately following most meals
- flatulence
- sense of fullness or nausea after eating
- itching around your rectum
- weak, peeling, cracked fingernails
- acne
- undigested food in the stool
- dilated capillaries on the face or rosacea

- iron deficiency
- chronic candida or parasites
- history of multiple food allergies
- acid reflux
- gastroesophageal reflux disease (GERD)
- a history of taking protein pump inhibitors, acid blockers or antacids

At one point I was able to check off at least five of these, which meant that I had low stomach acid and not enough digestive enzymes. In short, this meant that I was not properly digesting my food. This cartwheeled down my digestive tract, causing an overgrowth of bad bacteria in my small intestines and lending way to leaky gut, which, as we've already seen, contributes to autoimmune diseases and inflammation.

WAYS TO SUPPORT LOW STOMACH ACID

To naturally support low stomach acid, Dr. Bloom recommends fermented and cultured foods like kimchi, sauerkraut, fresh pickles, and some raw and sprouted vegetables as they naturally contain enzymes. Non-dairy cultured yogurt or kefir can also help as they contain beneficial bacteria.

To help stimulate stomach acid I took one tablespoon of apple cider vinegar or umeboshi plumb before each meal, especially before large meals that included a heavy protein. Ginger, gentian, and Swedish barks also help stimulate stomach acid production.

Another way to increase stomach acid is to supplement with betaine hydrochloric acid (HCL). Dr. Blum recommends starting with 250–350mg a day while eating, not before. Increase the dosage each day by one pill until reaching a maximum of eight pills. [8]

If you notice warmth or discomfort in your stomach right after eating then you've reached the maximum dosage. When you notice this, cut back one pill next time you eat until you reach a point where you have no discomfort. The higher the amount needed, the more severe the low stomach acid is.

Note: HCL should not be mixed with any other pain medications, including ibuprofen, acetaminophen, aspirin, etc.

BILE, DIGESTION, AND IMMUNITY

As my research broadened on the different parts of the amazing digestive process, I took notice of the next stop in the stream: your liver and the magical, bitter liquid it produces called bile.

Bile is a bitter fluid that is yellow, brown, or green in color. It has many important functions in your digestive process such as breaking down fat, calcium, and protein. Bile is needed to maintain normal fat levels in your blood, remove toxins from your liver, maintain proper acid/alkaline balance in your intestinal tract, and keep your colon from breeding harmful microbes.

Liver cells secrete bile into tiny canals called bile canaliculi, which eventually connect to your common bile duct, through which your liver supplies your gallbladder with the right amount of bile for digestion.

When the composition of your bile is not balanced, small cholesterol crystals begin to combine with other bile components to form tiny clots, which eventually clump together and become gallstones in your liver and gallbladder. Gallstones can obstruct your bile ducts, slowing down your liver. When these bile ducts are blocked, then bile production drops.

I learned a lot about the importance of bile from an Ayurvedic practitioner named Andreas Moritz. After overcoming a life in and out of the hospital, Andreas made the important connection with the health of your liver and healing. According to Andreas, to maintain a strong and healthy digestive system and feed your cells the right amount of nutrients, your liver should produce 1–1.5 quarts of bile per day.[9] Anything less will cause problems with digestion, elimination of waste, and detoxification of your blood.

It seems that most people have bile flow issues. This is evident in the large number of people who have their gallbladders surgically removed every day. With a congested liver and gallbladder, the bile gets thick and clumpy and doesn't flow well. Bile has to flow well to keep your intestines lubricated.

Your liver also connects to the pancreas via the common bile duct. The pancreas makes important enzymes that, along with bile, neutralize acid from your stomach. With thick bile your pancreas enzymes don't flow, which means your stomach acid is not neutralized. If there are not enough bile or pancreas enzymes, your stomach then dials down stomach acid to prevent burning a hole in your intestines. This means undigested food goes into your digestive tract. Again, this contributes to conditions like leaky gut.

WAYS TO IMPROVE BILE FLOW

There are several ways to help bile flow. It is recommended to drink a large glass of water 15–20 minutes before eating. This buffers your stomach lining so that it is hydrated and stimulates stomach acid production, signaling your body to produce more bile and enzymes to neutralize. Eating ginger before and during a meal also helps to trigger bile flow. Beets and cinnamon also get bile flowing.

The cellulose in leafy green vegetables attaches to your bile and helps escort it out of your body. If not enough vegetables are consumed then 93 percent of the bile is reabsorbed back into your liver, into your blood, causing damage to your arteries.

Eating good fats helps to slime up your liver and gallbladder to keep it functional. Otherwise, it dries up.

DO YOU HAVE ENOUGH GOOD GUYS IN YOUR GUT?

After the food you eat is or is not broken down and absorbed, it then travels through the vastness of your intestines. Within this large area of my body, my attention was brought to my gut flora, which is made up of trillions of microbe populations. These bugs in your gut nourish and balance your immune system. If your gut flora is off, then your whole system suffers.

There are three groups of gut flora:

- beneficial (anti-fungal, anti-microbial);
- opportunistic (fungi, protozoa, etc.); and
- transitional (go through us but don't settle, gathered from food and drink).

Beneficial microorganisms fight off the opportunistic microbes and prevent toxins from entering your system. If there are not enough good guys in the battle then the bad takes over, simple as that. If there are too many bad, opportunistic microbes, then your body does not absorb nutrients and things go haywire.

Unhealthy gut flora is developed at the start of life and relates to the mother. When the baby comes out of the mother's vagina at birth, it essentially swallows its batch of gut flora before entering the world. So if the mother's gut flora is off, then the baby's gut flora will be too. Babies that are delivered via C-section are filled with opportunistic microbes, since they were unable to swallow the beneficial microorganisms from their mother. Thus C-section babies are more likely to develop immune system deficiencies.

Breast-feeding is another essential piece in developing a healthy gut flora. Babies given formula and not breast-fed, or not breast-fed long enough, tend to have immune system issues too.

Later in life prescription medicines, especially antibiotics, throw off the balance of healthy gut flora. This is because antibiotics attack all microorganisms, including the good guys. Every dose of antibiotics opens up a window where pathogens are allowed in. This period can be two weeks or two months long.

Another factor is the tremendous amount of livestock in the United States that are fed antibiotics to ward off diseases associated with the awful practices in the industry. When we eat this meat those antibiotics enter our systems as well.

Birth control was another big contributor to my unhealthy gut flora as were over-the-counter, anti-inflammatory medications (NSAIDs).

In addition to all the pills, stress and toxins also affected the health of my gut flora. My prior diet high in refined carbohydrates, processed foods, and sugar only fed the bad guys in my gut.

HOW TO SUPPORT THE GOOD GUYS

According to Dr. Blum, there are specific foods that support the positive microorganisms in your gut and support healing the intestinal lining of your gut. These include:

- non-dairy yogurt
- non-dairy kefir
- fermented foods (like kimchi and sauerkraut)
- prebiotics, found in many vegetables and fiber
- ghee and coconut oil
- glutamine, found in animal protein, beans, cabbage, beets, spinach, and parsley

To help add to the good guys in your gut, a daily probiotic is also helpful as are digestive enzymes, which help to break down foods in your digestive tract. Once I added a good digestive enzyme into my regime, I noticed remarkable differences in my digestion.

FINAL STOP: THE COLON

The colon is the final step on our digestive journey. It is important for this pathway to remain clear so that bad bacteria won't pile up. A clogged colon is a breeding ground for toxic waste so it is important to have a couple of eliminations a day.

I learned that my poop is actually the most important indicator of my health and of how my body is functioning inside. Our stools are made up of about 75 percent water and the rest is a combo of fiber, mucus, and live and dead bacteria.

The bacteria in our stools come from the bugs in our digestive tract. As mentioned, having a healthy ratio of good bugs over bad is the key to good health. When the bad bugs outweigh the good then conditions like irritable bowel syndrome (IBS), colitis, and Crohn's disease come into play.

There are tests available that can measure the balance of good bacteria in our digestive tract through analysis of our poop. We can also evaluate the health of our digestive tract by simply examining the characteristics of our poop: its color, odor, shape, size, and even the sound it makes when it hits the water.

A healthy poop has the following characteristics:
- medium to light brown
- smooth and soft
- formed into one long shape, not a bunch of pieces
- about one to two inches wide and up to 18 inches long
- S-shaped, indicating a nice clearing of the lower intestine
- quietly and gently dives into the water
- not repulsively smelly
- uniform texture
- sinks slowly
- easy to pass, no strain or pain
- should be easy to clean off

Bright or black poop may indicate bleeding in your gastrointestinal tract. White, pale, or gray stools may indicate lack of bile. And yellow poop could indicate a giardia infection or gallbladder problem. Undigested food in your stool is an issue and as mentioned, is a symptom of low stomach acid. Increased mucus in the stool could indicate IBS, Crohn's Disease, colitis, or even colon cancer.

A poop with a really bad odor could mean your body is not absorbing nutrients correctly. Soft diarrhea often indicates food intolerances to lactose, artificial sweeteners, fructose, or gluten.

It takes an average body 18–72 hours to convert food into poop and pass it out of the body. Everyone is different and different factors can throw off bowel movements including diet, travel, medications, hormonal fluctuations, sleep patterns, exercise, illness, surgery, childbirth, and stress. But if there is less than one bowel movement happening in a day, then we have a problem!

WAYS TO PRODUCE A HEALTHY POOP

There are different things we can do to help improve the health of our poop and thus the health of ourselves.

- remove gluten
- eat whole foods
- avoid processed foods, more from the ground, less from a box
- avoid artificial sweeteners and excess sugar
- avoid chemical additives, including MSG
- avoid artificial coloring
- avoid excess caffeine
- add fermented foods to the diet
- add a good probiotic
- add digestive enzymes to help break down food
- increase fiber intake
- stay hydrated
- exercise, yoga does wonders for keeping poop moving

out!
- avoid pharmaceuticals
- manage stress

Don't forget to check your poop before you flush to see how your body reacts to certain foods and of how well your all-important digestive tract is flowing.

CLEARING THE COLON WITH COLONICS

I spent a good part of my 20s selling advertising over the phone to small businesses. One of my clients was under the category *colon hydrotherapy*, which made me chuckle. I had no idea what it actually was that they did at the time. The owner answered when I called one day and I ended up talking to her for a good amount of time. She was a certified colon hydrotherapist and I couldn't help but notice just how passionate she was about it.

She explained how colonics remove waste that gets stuck on the sides of the colon, things like pills, pesticides, and other chemicals that build up for years. By the end of the conversation my interest was piqued, but I wasn't quite ready to take the plunge. My biggest fear, I think, was having something up my butt. Ha.

It took me three years to finally do it. I made a last minute appointment so that I didn't have to stress and worry about the experience. I forced Ryan along with me for moral support. I went to a center that was close to our home. We were both so nervous sitting in the treatment area, staring at a large contraption called the Angel of Water. It was an open system, meaning the piece that is inserted was much smaller.

The colon hydrotherapist, Megan, was just as passionate as the woman I had spoken to years earlier. She showed us a video of how the whole process worked and made it seem super simple. It was weird at first, but as time moved on I got used to it. The water really helped to move out the stopped-up gunk and toxins that were stuck in my colon. I continued to get subsequent colonics as a detoxification method. Megan ended up becoming one of my good friends and the one that I could talk to about all the new things I was learning along my healing journey. Including the health and status of my poop!

The practice of colonics helped my body reduce bloating, constipation, and fatigue. I also found them to be very hydrating. *Note: As with any detoxification method, things are often a struggle before they get better. There may be initial detoxification reactions to colonics as old waste is finally cleared from the colon.*

EATING WITH DIGESTIVE RHYTHMS

In addition to what we eat, and how we eat, *when* we eat is important too. I learned about this important connection of biological digestive rhythms from an Ayurvedic practitioner by the name of John Douillard. He taught me that the body's digestive capacity is much lower in the morning and evening time, especially past 6:00 p.m., suggesting that these meals should be lighter. The production of bile and intestinal digestive juices actually peaks during midday, suggesting that the biggest meal of the day should be eaten at this time.

Thus, lunch should be the largest meal of the day. This important meal deserves our time and attention. According to John Douillard, "If the body is not satisfied at lunch, it will strain through the afternoon and crave an emotional meal or drink at night."[10]

After spending years in a corporate environment, I cut my lunches short so I could leave earlier. This meant that I was limited to a microwave and a half hour. Often times I'd just eat something small. If I did eat something substantial, my eating time was rushed so I could complete errands or some other project during this time. When I ate a light lunch, or a meal made up of all carbohydrates,

I'd crave sugar around 2:00–3:00 in the afternoon. If I didn't satisfy this craving, then it would extend into the night as after work to late night sugar binges.

Another eating pattern that can cause digestive issues and the formulation of gallstones in the liver and gallbladder is eating between meals. According to Ayurveda, eating before the previous meal has been digested is one of the major causes of illnesses.

In his book *3-Seasons Diet*, John Douillard writes:

> *The human digestive system is designed to eat a large meal and fully digest it before taking in substantially more. A large meal can take from one to three hours in the upper digestive tract. By eating small amounts throughout the day, we never give the digestive tract a rest. It is constantly engaged and this is unnatural for the body, which depends on cycles of rest and activity.*[11]

The interruption of snacks between meals forces your stomach to leave the previously eaten meal half-digested so that it can attend to the newly ingested food instead. This half digested food clogs up your colon, ferments, and putrefies causing toxins in the digestive tract, leading to further distress.

If your body is used to the practice of snacking between meals then it becomes conditioned and starts to expect these small feedings every couple of hours. If your body misses one of these mini-meals then blood sugar and energy levels drop and trigger a craving for emergency fuel in the way of carbohydrates or sugars. This causes an insulin response, resulting in peaks and valleys in blood sugar and a message to your body to save and store fat. Eating three solid meals a day helps create a steady energy flow and encourages your body to burn fat for fuel instead of glucose.

Once I shifted towards having lunch be my biggest, most protein-rich meal of the day—with breakfast and dinner being lighter in the way of soup, salad, juice, or fruit—I found that I felt better.

This cut back on the late afternoon crashes and sugar cravings I was accustomed to.

Not snacking between meals is hard, but I found that when I stopped this habit, I felt better too. My digestion improved significantly as did my energy levels. Changing my eating habits made a big difference in my overall health and healing. I started to become more in tune with how certain foods were making me feel and how significant shifts happened in my body when my digestive track had issues. Things were more smooth and in flow when this system was healthy and happy.

LESSON THREE: THE MONTHLY SYMPHONY

"Many women today refuse to remain ignorant. They are beginning to actively participate in all facets of their health care, enhancing their understanding of their fertility in the process."

~ Toni Weschler, Taking Charge of Your Fertility

THE SOMEDAYS

I learned to make the recommended dietary changes a part of my life since this really helped remove the pain that I was experiencing on a near daily basis and the digestive distress I'd experienced for much of my adult life. While I still had pretty painful periods, I appreciated that there were more days with little to no pain.

Ryan noticed the shifts in me too in more ways than one. My libido was warmly welcomed back by both of us. This was helpful on our new quest to make a baby. We both recognized that this could be the true ticket to me living a life free from the pain from endometriosis. While pregnancy isn't a sure fire bet to resolving endometriosis, I had met several women whose symptoms dissipated after having children. More importantly, we both felt ready to welcome a new child into our family.

So we got to work.

Months passed. Twelve cycles quickly added up to a year of no success. There were a handful of cycles where I was sure that I was pregnant. It's just one more ugly thing about endometriosis: the symptoms mimic those of pregnancy including sore boobs, nausea, emotional roller coasters, etc.

I would have these symptoms and they would bring with them the certainty that I was pregnant. That inevitably led to daydreaming and playing with all the what-ifs. What would we name him or her? How would my life change? In what month would the baby be born? Would he or she have my smile or Ryan's bright blue eyes?

On many occasions, I was unable to hold in my certainties and I would suggest to Ryan that it was possible I was pregnant. This would open up a whole new opportunity for excitement and imagination. I knew that Ryan really wanted to have a family and I knew that he would be the best father. I couldn't help but feel guilty for my broken womb. What if I was never able to have kids? I'd be crushing someone else's dream too.

Unable to stand the suspense, I would always end up buying a couple of pregnancy tests. But they were always negative. And usually within a day or two of taking them, my flow would appear more painful than ever, accompanied by feelings of disappointment, sadness, and failure. The painful contractions during these periods I envisioned similar to labor—a sick joke by the universe for a woman struggling with infertility. This pain cut deep in the very place where a new life grows.

At the end of all that pain there was no baby to show, only a stark emptiness. This pain was coupled with tears and emotional loss for a broken fantasy and the inevitable question: *Will it ever be me?*

Within this year of struggle I was invited to at least eight different baby showers. I went to one where half the party was pregnant! It was incredibly difficult for me to attend. My congratulations and forced smiles hid a reality I could not escape: something was wrong with me. A woman in her 30s with no children begs the question, "Well, when?"

"Someday," remained my reply, sometimes shakier than others.

Eventually I stopped attending the showers. I couldn't get over my own emotions tied to the occasion. More often than not I had to gulp back tears and suppress the emotions trying to play out on my face. I watched so many women I knew experience the beauty and wonder of growing a life inside of them. A life that would be born into the world and consume them with all the new experiences and firsts.

My heart ached.

I held onto doubts that I would ever be able to bear a child. My inability to be one of the moms became a lonely journey. On many occasions, I sat and listed to other moms talk about their kids. They presented questions that only other moms knew the answer to. I felt perpetually left out and alone.

When Ryan and I attended events together, our time was routinely spent watching young parents chasing after their kids. It presented us with an awkward situation that eventually led to us no longer getting invited anywhere. As the years passed, those in our circle of couple friends with no kids dwindled to a point of isolation.

The possibility of *never* was often to blame for my emotional turmoil. I was unable to see and accept someone else's happiness. I could only think of my own shortcomings. As each of my friends joined the mom club, there were fewer women around who were non-moms like me, fewer women who could relate to the pains associated with infertility.

Tension increased again between Ryan and I as did our mutual feelings of hate towards this disease that was standing in the way of bringing a new life into this world, a life that would reflect a little bit of each of us.

THE MAIN EVENT

As each month brought continued failure in me getting pregnant, I realized just how little I understood about the menstrual cycle and the changes that went on in my body each month. I had to admit that I had little idea how the whole pregnancy thing worked, and had always assumed that once I got off birth control and had unprotected sex that pregnancy would just happen.

In addition to my mother's brief conversation about the arrival of my monthly flow, I recalled that awkward fifth-grade conversation. You know the one, when the teachers separate all the girls from the boys for the first sex education lesson, which had included instruction about the woman's body and menstruation.

I walked away from those brief lessons with little knowledge about what actually happens during the menstrual cycle. I understood that the period was the main event and the different feminine products were presented in defense of this. The main question of the time was pad or tampon?

The whole process and related feminine products translated to shame for me. I asked my mother to buy my menstrual pads for me well into my teenage years. When I had to purchase them for myself, I was so embarrassed! I'd be sure to pick a checkout lane with a woman as I purchased other not-so-needed items so the pads wouldn't be the only thing waiting in plain view for everyone to see, an outward sign that I was bleeding.

When I used them, I was always sure to hide my feminine products and was extra careful not to rip off the wrapper too loudly, in fear that the woman in the next stall would hear me.

With the pain that accompanied my period and the focus and marketing dollars spent in promotion of this grand event, it made sense that my main focus of each month was menstruating. The problem was that I had never really learned what happened before that. Not until I realized that the before part was what I needed to worry about if I actually wanted to get pregnant.

THE WORKINGS OF THE MENSTRUAL CYCLE

After learning about my period as a young girl, the next phase of learning came in those awkward sex education classes as a teenager where focus shifted to different methods of protection so that you did not get pregnant and reasons why unprotected sex was dangerous. But there was still no mention as to how a woman could actually get pregnant. There was no mention of ovulation. The message was use a condom or birth control or you will get pregnant or catch something worse.

This lack of knowledge about my menstrual cycle was missing for much of my young adult life and made me rely on a doctor's knowledge to tell me about my body. I blindly followed the suggestion to take birth control without knowing what this choice actually did to the ebb and flow of my body's natural hormonal rhythms. I believed that by removing these pills from my body that I would just get pregnant.

Things were not that simple.

I'd been off of birth control for four years with no success in getting pregnant. As I traveled further down the road of infertility, I held strong to the notion that I did not want to resort to fertility drugs. I felt sure that my path of healing would eventually lead its way to pregnancy. The researcher in me believed that I would find a way to achieve this without more added hormones. That was when I came across Toni Weschler's book, *Taking Charge of Your Fertility*, which helped me gain knowledge about the workings of my cycle.

I wish that I'd been given this book at a much earlier age. It took three decades of life before I finally understood what happened each month during the whole menstrual cycle. This was important for me to understand because if I didn't know how it worked, then it was even more difficult to figure out how to fix it.

Toni's book taught me how to chart my menstrual cycle so I'd know what phase I was in and the times when I should be most fertile to achieve pregnancy. Charting my cycles helped me tune into the ebb and flow of the changes in my body and emotions each cycle and helped me find a much deeper connection between the troubles I was having with my menstrual cycle and certain markers that were off, namely progesterone.

I've provided a simplified breakdown of how the menstrual cycle works and the hormonal changes involved, in case you are in the dark like I was. If this is not new to you, then please feel free to skip ahead.

On a simple level, the whole purpose of your menstrual cycle is to prepare your body for pregnancy, whether you want it or not. The first half of your menstrual cycle is called your *follicular phase* and starts with follicular stimulating hormone (FSH). This hormone stimulates the maturity of 15–20 eggs in your ovaries. Each egg is enclosed in its own follicle that produces estrogen.

Estrogen is necessary for ovulation, which occurs when one ovary releases an egg from the most dominant follicle. This process takes anywhere from eight days to two weeks or more.

High levels of estrogen trigger a surge of luteinizing hormone (LH). This LH surge causes the egg to burst through your ovarian wall where it is picked up by finger-like projections of your fallopian tubes called fimbria, which pull the egg into one of your fallopian tubes.

After the egg is released from your ovary, the follicle that held it remains behind. It attaches to your interior ovarian wall and becomes a corpus luteum that starts to release progesterone.

The days following ovulation are called your *luteal phase*. Due to the fixed lifespan of your corpus luteum, the amount of days in this phase of your cycle should be consistent. Therefore, ovulation determines the length of your menstrual cycle. Your corpus luteum should have a life span of 12–16 days. Anything less than this amount of time indicates there are issues with your progesterone levels.

If fertilization of your egg does not occur, then levels of progesterone eventually drop, signaling to the body to break down the corpus luteum. When this happens menstruation begins, indicating the start of a new cycle. With menstruation, the lining of your uterus is shed.

If your egg is fertilized and pregnancy happens, then your corpus luteum hangs around into the beginning of pregnancy. It continues to secrete progesterone to help maintain your uterine lining for eight to ten weeks, after which the placenta takes over progesterone production.

Occasionally your ovaries may not release an egg at all and ovulation does not happen. This is termed anovulation and is common when cysts are on your ovaries. Follicular cysts happen in the first half of your cycle and are often stimulated by high insulin levels from consuming too many foods with a high glycemic load. Anovulation is also a common occurrence with women with polycystic ovary syndrome (PCOS). If you don't ovulate then there is no chance for pregnancy.

So that's the basic hormonal symphony of your menstrual cycle. I hope you learned something new. Knowledge is power.

CHARTING THE MENSTRUAL CYCLE

As I alluded to earlier in this chapter, one thing that really helped me connect with the ebb and flow of my menstrual cycle was with the simple action of charting my cycle. By doing this, I was able to figure out the patterns of my cycle and begin deciphering what had, for years, been a mystery to me. It also provided me with evidence of the workings of my body that I could share with other health practitioners in a traditional medical setting if, by chance, they were educated in this practice. And of course, it gave me something to share with alternative wellness practitioners like my acupuncturist.

This powerful method is an easy way to gain feedback into your own cycle, whether you are trying to get pregnant or not get pregnant without the aid of birth control, or if you are trying to figure out what's wrong within your menstrual cycle. By charting my monthly cycle I was able to detect that I had progesterone issues visible by my short luteal phase of only 9–10 days, when it should have been 12–16 days. I also learned that my waking body temperature tended to be higher than what is considered normal. This prompted me to test my thyroid. I found out that I had Hashimoto's,[iii] a condition that can affect body temperature.

Here are the basic steps on how to get started on charting your own menstrual cycle, but this is only the tip of the iceberg. I highly recommend the book *Taking Charge of Your Fertility* by Toni Weschler for a more thorough explanation of how to chart your cycle and how to decipher your body's messages from this graphical explanation.

To further assist in charting your cycle, I also suggest using a secondary charting application. I use the free charting service tied into Toni Weschler's book at www.tcoyf.com. Another popular app is Fertility Friend at www.fertilityfriend.com.

STEP ONE: TAKE NOTE OF YOUR WAKING (BASAL BODY) TEMPERATURE

Take note of your waking body temperature each morning as soon as you get up, before doing anything. If you can take it while you are still in bed, even better.

Try and take your temperature at the same time every morning, give or take an hour. You can take your temperature orally or vaginally, so long as you remain consistent.

If you take your temperature at a different time or if there is some other factor that could impact your body temperature (stress, illness, travel or moving), you should note that information. The later into the day you take your temperature, the warmer it will be.

There are additional factors that can increase your waking temperatures such as:

- having a fever;
- drinking alcohol the night before;

iii   Hashimoto's disease, also known as chronic lymphocytic thyroiditis, is a condition in which your immune system attacks your thyroid gland. The resulting inflammation often leads to an underactive thyroid gland (hypothyroidism).

- getting less than three hours of consecutive sleep before taking it;
- taking it at a substantially different time than usual; and
- using an electric blanket or heating pad that you don't normally use.

If you wake up earlier than the time you've set to take it, then it is suggested to adjust your temperature by a tenth of a degree for each half hour earlier than your set time. For example, if you normally take your temperature at 7:00 a.m. and you wake up half an hour earlier, then you would subtract one-tenth of a degree (0.1) from your daily temperature.

Similarly, if you wake up later than your set time then you would add one-tenth of a degree (0.1) to your daily temperature for each half-hour. For example, if you normally take your temperature at 7:00 a.m. and wake up an hour later at 8:00 a.m., then you would add two tenths of a degree (0.2).

According to Toni Weschler, pre-ovulatory temperatures typically range from 97–97.7 degrees Fahrenheit (36.1-36.5 degrees Celsius), with post-ovulatory temperatures rising to about 97.8 degrees Fahrenheit (or 36.3 degrees Celsius) and higher. If you have waking body temperatures that are consistently low (97.3 or lower in the pre-ovulatory stage) then this could be indicative of an underactive thyroid.

Temperatures rise within a day or so after ovulation, the result of the heat-inducing hormone, progesterone. Pre-ovulatory temperatures are suppressed by estrogen. After ovulation, temperatures should remain elevated until your next period, about 12–16 days later.

Waking temperatures can be helpful in predicting how long the menstrual cycle will be, as it can identify a delayed ovulation. Once the temperature rises, the days to follow tend to be a consistent number. Normally menstruation follows 12–16 days after the temperature shift.

The cover line. Remember that after ovulation, temperatures should quickly rise above the range of low temperatures that precede it. This thermal shift is often so obvious that you should be able to spot it by glancing at the chart. However, in order to interpret it accurately, you want to draw a cover line to help you differentiate between low, pre-ovulatory temperatures and high, post-ovulatory temperatures.

If you use software at www.tcoyf.com or www.fertilityfriend.com to help chart your cycle it will help you determine your cover line. If you choose to chart on paper or with different graphing software, like Microsoft Excel, then you need to learn how to detect your cover line.

1. After your period ends, as you are charting your temperatures, always notice the highest of the previous six days.

2. Identify the first day your temperature rises at least two-tenths of a degree above the highest temperature.

3. Go back and highlight the last six temperatures before the rise.

4. Draw the cover line one-tenth of a degree above the highest of that cluster of six highlighted days preceding the rise.

If you have occasional high temperatures that are artificially high, you may cover the outlying temperatures with your thumb when you are determining your cover line.

STEP TWO: OBSERVE YOUR CERVICAL FLUID

Charting your daily temperatures helps determine when you ovulated, but it is not as helpful in determining when you are going to ovulate. For this, it is helpful to evaluate your daily cervical fluid. A general pattern of cervical fluid from the end of menstruation until your next period is as follows: dry -> sticky -> creamy -> egg white/

slippery -> nothing/dry/sticky.

As ovulation approaches, your cervical fluid should get increasingly wet. When the body is really fertile (near ovulation) then it should secrete a larger amount of fluid that may be very wet and/or like raw egg whites. This may be extremely slippery or even stretch. It's usually clear or partially streaked, but it can be yellow, pink, or red tinged. A lot of time this fertile fluid will leave a fairly symmetrical round pattern of fluid on your underwear due to its high water content.

The most important factor of this extremely fertile cervical fluid is its lubricative quality. A trick to help you identify the actual quality of the cervical fluid is to notice what it feels like to run tissue or your finger across your vaginal lips. Does it feel dry, impeding movement? Is it smooth? Or does it simply glide across? As you approach ovulation, this movement should glide easily. It should have a slippery sensation. Be sure to check when you're not sexually aroused, as this can alter cervical fluid.

Try to check cervical fluid every time you use the bathroom. Doing vaginal contractions called Kegels can help to get the cervical fluid to flow down to the opening. Cervical fluid is most likely to flow out after a bowel movement.

Other signs of pending ovulation include mid-cycle spotting, pain near the ovaries, an increase in sex drive, bloating, water retention, and breast tenderness. Ovulation is the time when estrogen peaks, which means that it can bring pain, especially for women who have endometriosis.

Right after your period you will likely have a "dry spell." Following ovulation estrogen drops off and the cervical fluid dries up. The lack of cervical fluid will usually last until the end of the cycle. Some women may notice a very wet, watery sensation prior to menstruation. This is due to the drop in progesterone that precedes the breaking up of the corpus luteum. This could change from month to month. Your particular cycle patterns will have their own unique development.

Note your cervical fluid in your charting software, or if you are keeping track by hand then input these observances into a journal.

The discovery of the connection between cervical fluid and ovulation was a pretty big revelation for me. I realized again just how little I knew about my menstrual cycle. With the extra cream in my panties I thought I was getting recurring infections! Little did I know that this was completely normal.

It took me a couple of cycles of charting to get a better understanding of the characteristics of my own cycle. I found it helpful to also note other symptoms felt during each day of the cycle, both physically and emotionally. This gave some sense to the twinges and pains that happened mid-cycle as ovulation occurred and the stressed out and anxiety ridden emotions that were common for me prior to ovulation and the start of my period.

Once I understood what was going on, I felt a renewed sense of power over this magical symphony inside of me.

LESSON FOUR: HORMONES, ENDOMETRIOSIS & FERTILITY

"The most common treatment for endometriosis, once diagnosed, is hormone therapy... the problem with these approaches is that they don't really cure the disease, they simply shut down the hormonal stimulation of it for a while."

~ Christiane Northrup, Women's Bodies, Women's Wisdom

BETTER TO HAVE LOVED AND LOST

In the summer of my 31st year, I decided to stop obsessing about getting pregnant. In fact, I made the decision to *not* get pregnant. This decision lifted such stress from me. I knew in my heart that someday we would have a child, but I was tired of obsessing about it. So instead of rejoicing when Ryan and I made love on ovulation day, I felt content when we didn't. It removed the hope and disappointment of possibility.

Fast forward to Halloween 2013. Growing up it was my favorite holiday. I enjoyed dressing up and having the chance to be someone or something else for a day. As an adult, however, I spent that Halloween in my everyday clothes in my cubicle at work. I was plain old me.

On a routine trip to the ladies' room that day, I was met with a surprise. With a wipe of the toilet paper came a creamy ovulation-like fluid. I found this odd, especially since I was eleven days past ovulation. As I made my way back to my desk, I was stopped by one of my co-workers.

"I have a confession to make," she said, "I've had dreams about you the past couple of nights."

"What about?" I asked.

She drew an arc in front of her belly. "You were pregnant."

"Really?"

Hmmm. I had not shared my fertility issues with her.

A nearby co-worker piped in and asked, "Do you want to have children?"

"I do, but I have some fertility issues."

I found it easier to put that fact out there. It saved having to hear the same question over and over, the question that always stirred up something painful inside of me.

I returned to my desk and was a bit distraught. First the odd cream in the bathroom then my co-worker's out-of-the-blue comment that she'd been dreaming about me. I'd reached a point in my life where I knew synchronicities like these meant something.

I did some Goggling about the out of place cervical fluid so late past ovulation. Sure enough, I found that it could be a sign of early pregnancy. In review of my basal body temperatures for the month, I was only further reassured that this could be a possibility. In fact, my temps looked the best they had all year.

I'd pushed aside thoughts of pregnancy and had made a decision to stop trying. The stress from all of it was too much and the disappointment with the arrival of my period each month slowly chipped away at my heart. But being that it was Halloween, I made a different decision. If I could be anything I wanted for just one day, this year I was going to be pregnant. The thought made me smile.

These thoughts didn't leave my mind in the days that followed as my daily temperatures remained high and my luteal phase extended longer than I'd seen it all year. To put my mind at ease, I picked up a pregnancy test.

Ryan shook his head. "Don't get your hopes up."

I had butterflies in my stomach as I took a trip to our upstairs bathroom to take the test. I peed on the white stick, slipped on the plastic cover, and set it on a sheet of toilet paper next to me. I was pretty sure that I knew the answer. I felt different this time. My intuition knew it to be true. As expected, the little round window showed two pink lines, though the positive side was a little lighter.

I stared at the result for a long time and the butterflies did flips in my tummy. With wobbly knees I made my way back downstairs to tell Ryan the news.

My big smile gave it away before I told him, "As expected."

He returned my beaming expression, "What?"

"It's still very early. But yes!"

I couldn't sleep that night. My mind was filled with possibility amidst an underlying worry: was it going to stick?

I knew from my interactions with other women with endometriosis that miscarriages were a common occurrence. I also knew from charting my cycle for nearly a year that I likely had progesterone issues. My luteal phase only ranged, on average, 9–10 days.

When I learned that I was pregnant I continued to take my morning temperatures. I wanted to make sure it remained high and each morning it did, I breathed a sigh of relief—until the morning that it dropped.

I shoved the thermometer in the drawer and stared at my pale reflection in the mirror, into my own scared eyes. A moment later my fears seemed to be confirmed when I discovered a swipe of pink blood on the toilet paper. That vision of pink blood pushed me over the edge. This was it. I couldn't escape the signs; a miscarriage was on the way.

I spent another day in my cubicle at work doing compulsive Google searches about miscarriage signs, escaping in between to drop some tears in the bathroom stall. My boss spotted my puffy, tear-stained face and immediately asked me what was wrong.

"I think I'm going to lose it," I whispered.

I fought back another wave of tears that I'd somehow managed to get under control only a moment before. She assured me that spotting early on was normal. In fact, it had happened to her and she went on to have a healthy baby girl.

My Google searches taught me that temperatures could be all over the place during pregnancy, so it was best to stop temping once receiving a positive pregnancy test or you may drive yourself crazy. I took a deep breath and tried to be optimistic, but I couldn't shake my sinking suspicion.

When the spotting returned the next day, my heart sank even

further. I made an appointment to see my primary doctor the next morning, since I couldn't get in to see a gynecologist, and said some prayers. I woke the next day with a familiar twinge in my uterus, one that I knew all too well.

Flow was coming.

I made a desperate cry to the support group that I was part of and was met with a choir of positive responses: spotting was normal in early pregnancy and pain was also normal with endometriosis and pregnancy.

Ryan drove me to the appointment, as I was in a lot of pain. The doctor checked my blood levels and told me she'd have the results the next day. When I got home the pain accelerated. I was having constant contractions from my uterus and this pain was cascading throughout my body. I rolled in a ball and let out a hum of moans.

When I later saw the toilet full of blood, I knew it was over. Yet I held onto the possibility that this could be normal, especially since I hadn't seen any large clots come out. With my last sliver of hope that I was still pregnant, I refrained from taking any pain medication and went to bed that night in horrible pain. The only way I was able to get to sleep was with a simple one-word mantra that I repeated over and over with energy and focus on my trembling uterus: *calm*.

When I finally fell asleep I dreamed of my grandmother, who had passed away nearly a year earlier. She was a younger version of herself, as I'd known her as a child. She reached out to me and retrieved a white light from my hands. When I woke up the next morning I passed what I believe was the physical start to our child's life. I stared at the ball of tendon-looking mass for a while before flicking the handle to the toilet, granting a small goodbye.

The spasms stopped and I knew it was over.

LIFE AFTER DEATH

Later that day I made a trip to the gynecologist's office dressed in my sagging black sweats and sweatshirt. I took a seat next to Ryan in the waiting room and did my best to keep from screaming, the pain in my pelvic region was that intense.

It took longer than usual for the women at the front desk to acknowledge our existence before sending me to pee in a cup. I held up the cup when I was done and saw big red clots floating in it. I dumped it out into the toilet and tried again without much success. Not knowing what else to do, I placed the plastic cup filled with red in the metal box on the wall and quickly shut the door.

After returning to the waiting room, I was soon greeted by a young, smiling woman. I couldn't force the edges of my mouth to rise to meet hers. Instead, I scuffled behind her into the ultrasound examination room. I cringed when she told me that she was going to do a vaginal ultrasound.

I bit my lip when she popped the white wand inside of me and moved it around my pulsating insides. I felt each move she made, saying silent prayers for it soon to be over. Ryan sat silent next to me, shaken too by the day's events. The technician told me that she did not see anything left in my uterus and confirmed that what I had experienced was likely a miscarriage.

Then we were led and left in a small, cold, white room with a single round table and three chairs. In the middle of the table was a box of tissues.

I thought, *Seriously? Is this where they send all the miscarriages?* I sent a knowing glance Ryan's way.

A young woman with mousy brown hair entered the room and reached out her hand to shake mine. She sat down and asked me to explain what had happened. She nudged the tissues my way.

I swallowed down tears, but they only pooled up deeper when she said the key phrase, "It's not your fault."

She told me that it was normal to go back over every detail of the pregnancy in review of what had gone wrong, but that in all reality miscarriages were a common thing. Even though it isn't really talked about, she said that most women go through it.

"I need to do an examination," she said, pushing back her chair.

An exam? I followed after her into an examination room and quickly got undressed. I was so tired of sitting and bleeding on paper-lined tables. My insides ached from the ultrasound as my uterus continued to burst out in spasms.

When she returned to the room she asked me to relax my legs out and before I knew it, I had a pair of cold clamps shoved inside of me. I slid up the examination table and cried out in pain. Tears streamed down my cheeks.

"I don't understand why this is necessary," I cried.

"I just have to make sure that everything came out," she said.

She reached inside of me and pulled at whatever was already on its way out. She closed her fist around it and held it away.

"You don't need to see this," she said, disposing of whatever it was into a metal trashcan.

I stared at the closed trash bin in silent horror and flinched in pain as she pulled the clamps out of me. I fought back the urge to kick the nurse in the face and pulled my legs together.

"I'm ready to go now," I said in a quiet, firm tone.

I tuned out any other words she told me. The pain inside resonated with anger. With a solemn, tear streaked face I made my way out of the doctor's office with my head down. I felt empty, broken.

In the nights that followed, I did exactly what the nurse had told me not to do. I replayed the things that could have impacted a failed pregnancy. Was it stress? Low progesterone? Was my body not ready? I passed through many of the stages of grief for a lost loved one: shock, anger, denial, and depression. I developed a hatred for my body and quickly slipped back into thoughts of not being good enough. And I filled myself up with sweets, French fries, and red wine.

My heart hurt as it held on to a deep loss that reflected in the shine of a newborn's eyes. I couldn't help but think, *What if?*

Eventually I made it to acceptance. I thought it a positive sign that I was able to get pregnant. Something finally connected and I was not ready to lose hope that it would not connect again.

BALANCING PROGESTERONE AND ESTRADIOL

As was natural for me, I went back into research mode. What was going on with my hormones? I reached a better understanding about the hormonal havoc that is common with endometriosis and related infertility with the interplay of the two primary hormones in the menstrual cycle: progesterone and estrogen.

I was able to better grasp the significant relationship between these two main hormones by reading writings from Dr. John Lee. He was an international authority and pioneer in natural hormone balance as he dedicated his life to helping women achieve this. He published many conclusions about the negative consequences of synthetic hormones. Even though he died in October of 2003, his books remain best-selling sources of information on how to obtain a balance between progesterone and estrogen.

Progesterone is a steroid hormone made by the ovaries when your body ovulates. It is also made in smaller amounts by your adrenal glands and in even smaller amounts by some nerve cells. It is manufactured in your body from a steroid hormone called pregnenolone and is a precursor to most other steroid hormones. Progesterone helps the female body regulate menstrual cycles. It is essential for creating and maintaining pregnancy and low progesterone can cause miscarriages.

The ovaries produce three different types of estrogen: estrone, estradiol, and estriol. Estrone and estradiol are the most concentrated and therefore the most potent. They stimulate cell growth of the uterine lining in your body's preparation for pregnancy during each menstrual cycle.

In excess, estrone and estradiol are bad because they stimulate cell growth, including cancer cell growth especially in the breasts and reproductive organs. They also feed endometrial cell growth in the case of endometriosis.

Progesterone is very important because it does the opposite of estradiol.

Endometriosis is most commonly an estrogen dominant condition, meaning there is not enough progesterone to balance the effects of estrogen. Estrogen dominance comes from not having enough progesterone or from having too much estrogen. In his book, *Hormone Balance Made Easy*, Dr. John Lee provides symptoms of an imbalance in either of these key hormones:[12]

Symptoms of low progesterone include:

- PMS
- insomnia
- early miscarriage
- painful or lumpy breasts
- unexplained weight gain
- cyclical headaches
- anxiety
- infertility
- hot flashes and night sweats

Symptoms of excess estrogen include:

- puffiness, bloating
- cervical dysplasia (abnormal pap smear)

- rapid weight gain
- breast tenderness
- heavy bleeding
- mood swings
- anxiety
- depression
- migraines (especially premenstrual)
- headaches
- insomnia
- foggy thinking
- red flush on the face
- gallbladder problems
- weepiness
- aches and pains
- allergies
- fatigue
- hair loss
- memory loss
- night sweats
- oversensitivity
- PMS

Wow. The list for estrogen dominance is *really* long. This estrogen dominance problem also contributes to fibroids, glandular dysfunction, and depression. If you look around, it is evident that these conditions are afflicting growing numbers of women. It is easy to see why having a proper amount of progesterone to balance all the estrogen is a key and why eliminating excess estrogens from the body is important.

According to Dr. John Lee, the best way to test for hormonal imbalances is through the saliva. You may purchase self-administered saliva tests on his web site at www.johnleemd.com.

The best time to test progesterone/estradiol levels is on the seventh day past ovulation, when progesterone should peak. A healthy ratio of progesterone to estradiol is at least 200 to 1.

Dr. John Lee is a strong proponent for the use of progesterone cream. He also advises the use of bio-identical progesterone cream, which is specifically designed to work with your individual body. This can be obtained by prescription from a compounding pharmacy.

Additional factors affecting a hormonal imbalance between progesterone and estrogen can include diet, poor sleep, excessive alcohol use, smoking, and birth control. Poor stress management can also be a huge factor.

ESTROGEN IN THE ENVIRONMENT

Unfortunately, a lot of the imbalances in bad estrogens come from the environment, so they are harder to avoid. These chemical imitators are called xenoestrogens. They are considered environmental estrogens and are synthetic substances that, when absorbed in the body, function similarly to estradiol, the bad estrogen. These chemical imitators of estrogen interfere with the action and/or production of our natural hormones and fuel the growth of endometriosis. They can also increase breast cancer growth. Xenoestrogens are easily absorbed through your skin. They implant themselves into the tissue of your body and the residue remains in your body for years after exposure, as they are difficult to detoxify through your liver.

Xenoestrogens are found in:

- pesticides sprayed on our foods;
- phthalates found in plastics and personal care products;
- bisphenoal a (BPA) found in hard plastics and the lining of cans;
- noylphenol found in cleaning products;
- estrogen-based birth control pills;

- estrogen-based hormone replacement therapy (HRT);
- polychlorinated biphenyls (PCBs) found in plastics, paints, etc.;
- dioxins often found in the meat of conventionally farmed animals;
- benzoapyrene found in sun blocks, perfumes, soaps, and printer toner;
- heavy metals including lead, mercury, and cadmium; and
- parabens found in most cosmetics and beauty products.

Below are some recommendations to help avoid further consumption of xenoestrogens.

- Avoid non-organic meat and animal products as these animals are fed hormones to speed their time to market. Also, hormones are used to plump the cattle to produce an animal that will retain water so that when cooked the meat is more tender and succulent.
- Eat organic foods as much as possible to limit exposure to pesticides.
- Do no heat up plastics and eat or drink from them. This includes plastic bottles that have been in the sun.
- Use glass or ceramic to eat off of and to store food.
- Use natural laundry detergents and avoid fabric softeners, as these put petrochemicals right on your skin.
- Update all beauty products and everything that comes in contact with your skin to eliminate toxic chemicals. Keep close attention on removing products that contain parabens.
- Update cleaning products to natural solutions. Both lemon and apple cider vinegar are great natural cleaning agents.
- Stop taking birth control with synthetic estrogens that

contributes further xenoestrogens in your body.

- Use a good water filter and remove any mercury fillings from your mouth.

I updated everything that came in contact with my skin in hopes of avoiding these environmental estrogens. One of my favorite additions into my beauty and cleaning regime was Castile soap. This natural soap makes a great base for body wash, hand soap, and cleaning products.

Another thing that I updated was my menstruation pads. The conventional commercial, chemically ridden, bleached pads add additional toxins at an entry point to our delicate reproductive organs. Conventional tampons have also been linked to dioxin toxicity, which has links to endometriosis. Instead, I've opted for organic cotton pads. One more option to consider is menstrual cups. These do not contain the chemicals you pick up from conventional pads and tampons. While I haven't tried this option personally, I know a lot of ladies who love them.

To help move out xenoestrogens picked up in the body, deep detoxification is suggested with the primary focus being on your liver and colon.

Also helpful is including a good amount of cruciferous vegetables in the diet. These include cabbage, broccoli, kale, cauliflower. Cruciferous vegetables help break down bad estrogens so they can exit the body.

Remember that if you have thyroid issues then it is best to eat cruciferous vegetables lightly cooked or steamed.

Another option to help move out excess estrogen is to supplement with calcium-D-glucarate, a botanical extract found in grapefruit, apples, oranges, broccoli, spinach, and Brussels sprouts.

Xenoestrogens are all around us and if you don't pay attention, it is very easy to come in contact with way too many of them. The good news is that by following the strategies in this chapter, it is possible to avoid a lot of them. I do believe that these changes have had a positive impact on my pain levels. By clearing out the xenoestrogens and related toxins from my personal environment, I was able to stop adding fuel to the fire.

REGRETS OF LONG TERM BIRTH CONTROL EFFECTS

Looking back it is obvious that the biggest source of xenoestrogens collected in my body was the decade of estrogen-based birth control pills I took. In all the years that I popped those little white birth control pills, not once did I stop to think about the impact they were having on my body. I just knew that they somehow kept me from getting pregnant and that they kept the pain from my endometriosis at bay. So I continued to take them, with little consideration of the long-term effects.

In her book, *Women's Bodies, Women's Wisdom*, Dr. Christiane Northrup says:

> But pills don't heal anything; they simply mask the underlying issues in the body or put an imbalance to sleep for a while. Taking birth control pills to regulate a woman's period is like shooting out the indicator light on the dashboard of your car that tells you that the engine needs attention.[13]

Once I stopped putting these artificial hormones into my body, I faced the reality of these side effects and couldn't help but wonder if this so called birth control had become a permanent thing. Birth control prevents pregnancy by stopping the body from ovulating. When there is no ovulation, there cannot be a pregnancy. When the body does not ovulate, it also fails to produce progesterone because without ovulation there is no development of a corpus luteum, which is responsible for progesterone production.

Birth control essentially turns off the body's own hormone production and replaces it with synthetic hormones. I started taking the pill when I was 17 years old, a time of my life when my body was still maturing. Then for the ten years after that, I essentially turned off my body's natural hormone rhythms. In short, my body was not producing progesterone for a decade, during what should have been the most fertile period of my life. Moving forward into my thirties at a lowered fertility time, I wondered if my body even knew how to produce progesterone?

In addition to turning off my progesterone production, the birth control pills had also stripped my body of essential nutrients including B vitamins, folic acid, vitamin C, magnesium, and zinc. These nutrients support antioxidant activity and demonstrate anti-inflammatory effects. B vitamins are needed for ovarian hormones and a lack in these essential vitamins is a big component in infertility. In addition, I learned that B vitamins support the liver. They also enrich the lining of the uterus and support adrenal functioning. B vitamins are also necessary for the formulation of progesterone and serotonin. For ten long years, I took those little white pills with little reconciliation for the essential vitamins I was losing.

In retrospect, the decision to take birth control for such a long time was not a good choice. If I could go back with the knowledge that I gained much later in life about natural methods of healing then I would have never, ever have put those little white pills into my body. But I am unable go back. Instead, I have worked on letting go of this regret, simply because I can't allow it to forever continue nagging at my thoughts.

I understand that the decision to take birth control is tricky for some women, as it is often presented as one of the main methods of treating endometriosis. When I stopped taking it, my gynecologist continued to push it on me every single time I saw her. It seemed to be the accepted choice, with few willing to question the impacts.

And while it came with many side effects, it did help ease the pain from my periods. With this came a dilemma. I wanted the pain to go away and birth control pills were a quicker fix. The natural way required much more patience, within which were times where I had to endure pain. That being said, I was ignorant about how the pill worked and just how impactful that choice would have on my future hormonal health. My hope is that by sharing this information with you, it will make you think twice about starting or continuing to take birth control pills.

If you do decide to stop taking the pill, then be aware that you will likely experience side effects as your natural hormones work to wake up again and your body works to remove the pill's artificial hormones.

LESSON FIVE: CLEAR DETOXIFICATION PATHWAYS

"If you live in today's environment but never pay attention to good detoxification, you end up like a tree that has been growing by a busy highway for years, absorbing smog, dirty water and the stress of loud cars going by. You end up polluted and wilted, with dull, spindly leaves and stunted roots."

Alejandro Junger, Clean

TREADING THROUGH THE TOXINS

Once I started paying attention to all the toxins in my environment and the xenoestrogens that were contributing to the excess estrogen load in my body, I started to feel quite overwhelmed. I recognized that these toxicities were relevant in the production and pain of endometriosis, as these toxins taxed my detoxification pathways, which were responsible for moving out excess estrogens that fed endometriosis.

Toxins prevented my body from functioning properly. Toxins that were stored in my body eventually overwhelmed my liver and re-entered my system to be stored in my cells and tissues. That toxic overload caused inflammation in my body and eventually led to Hashimoto's.

I learned just how sensitive the endocrine system is to toxins in the environment, especially the thyroid. It is no wonder thyroid disease has become almost a normalcy among the women that I meet.

While the diet changes that I made helped me with the daily, chronic pain, I was still experiencing painful periods that were knocking me off of my feet. After learning about the impacts of toxins in my body, I came to believe that the persistent pain with my periods could be a result of toxic overload in my body.

If I was going to overcome this I needed to first get away from adding a deeper toxic burden to my body. It became a constant battle to avoid the chemicals and poisons readily presented in our food and products offered for everyday sale, in the air we breathe, the water we bathe in.

After going through a phase of freak-out about all these toxins, I came to the understanding that I was not going able to avoid all of them 100 percent. I did my best with my individual consumption. The products and foods in my home were as chemically absent as possible, but my home was only a small space amidst the toxic landscape. I worked in a corporate job where I was away from home 40 hours a week. I couldn't help but notice the multiple times a day I washed my hands with the provided soap in the bathrooms, soap that was likely filled with toxins, seeping into my skin every hour.

Thus, I became the odd one who started to bring my own natural soap each time I went to the bathroom. Ha.

My next line of defense was with the improvement of my body's detoxification channels. Much of this started with shifts in my diet, which helped move things out of my colon. I learned that a clogged colon must be cleared first before moving to deeper cleansing programs. After getting this under control my focus shifted to the other detoxification channels including my lymphatic system, skin, lungs, kidneys, and almighty liver.

THE LYMPHATIC SYSTEM'S ROLE IN HEALING

I first gained knowledge about the importance of a well-functioning lymphatic system from Ayurvedic practitioner, Dr. John Douillard. His teachings really helped me get on track to a new level of healing. I learned that the lymphatic system is the largest circulatory system in my body and is made up of anywhere from 600–800 lymph nodes spread out in my body.

The lymph system picks up fluids and waste products from the spaces between our cells and filters and cleans them then transports to our blood for elimination in a process known as lymphatic drainage. The problem is, this system is easily clogged up from the many toxins and stress in our environment. When our lymphatic system is not working properly, waste and toxins build up in our bodies causing inflammation and disease.

One theory as to how endometriosis spreads is through our lymphatic system. This makes sense considering that our reproductive organs drain into our lymphatic system. If this system is clogged then parts of our endometrium could end up in places they don't belong.

Our lymphatic system is closely tied to our circulatory and urinary systems. The final waste products are released out of our kidneys in our urine.

How had I not learned about this important system sooner?

Turns out our lymphatic system is generally overlooked in Westernized medicine until it is too late and things like cancer take hold. Too much focus is spent on the health of our blood, which in fact is a direct reflection of the health of our lymphatic system.

According to Dr. John Douillard, many of the symptoms related to endometriosis were actually signs of a backed up lymphatic system, including: [14]

- painful, irregular, heavy, or missing periods;
- swollen/tender breasts prior to menstruation;
- skin issues such as breakouts and eczema;
- intestinal issues such as bloating, constipation and diarrhea;
- fatigue;
- allergies;
- joint pain;
- headaches;
- cellulite; and
- swollen glands.

Dr. Douillard explained that our lymphatic system is like the drain in our body. If the drain get back up then gunk gets stuck and builds up in our body. There are natural ways to help get our lymphatic system moving.

- Sipping warm water every 10 minutes, every day for two weeks. The hot water dilates our cells and keeps our lymph nodes open so they are better able to clear out.

- Drinking plenty of water at room temperature each day. Water helps clear out our "drains."
- Eat a diet made of 60–70 percent alkaline foods. This reduces inflammation in our body and helps keep our lymphatic system healthy. Most fruits and vegetable are super alkalizing. Leafy greens are a great choice.
- Dry skin brush. This helps remove old skin and the brushing movement helps move our lymph. Simply brush your skin prior to showering in the direction of your heart. The lymph system sits right under the skin level, so you don't need to brush hard.
- Frequent massages help clear out toxins from our lymphatic system. There is a specific type called lymphatic drainage massage that helps to increase flow of our lymphatic system. It removes waste at the cellular level and assists in bringing oxygen and nutrients to our cells. Lymphatic drainage can be especially helpful when healing from surgery (wait at least six weeks after surgery to get one).
- Jumping on a mini trampoline or jump rope are both said to stimulate lymphatic flow.
- The Ayurvedic herb manjistha is said to support natural functioning of the lymphatic system. It purifies our blood and detoxifies our thyroid.
- Frequent sauna visits help clear out toxins through our skin, and keep our lymphatic system from getting backed up.

CASTOR OIL AND LYMPHATIC FLOW

Another option that helps to stimulate lymphatic flow are castor oil packs. Castor oil comes from a plant native to India. It has been used for a very long time for various ailments. It is antiviral, antibacterial, and anti-fungal.

When applied to your skin the oil diffuses into your body and stimulates internal movement. When applied to your skin castor oil helps:

- increase circulation of blood and lymph;
- decrease pain;
- improve digestion;
- uterine fibroids;
- ovarian cysts;
- headaches and migraines;
- constipation and other intestinal disorders; and
- gallbladder and liver conditions.

Castor oil packs boosts our immune system by improving function of our thymus gland, which produces lymphocytes, the immune system's disease fighting cells stored mainly in our lymphatic tissue— thymus gland, spleen and lymph nodes. Increasing lymphocytes remove toxins at a faster rate from our body. This promotes overall healing.

Castor oil should be pretty easy to find. Check your local health food store. If you can find organic, that is the best choice.

HOW TO MAKE A CASTOR OIL PACK

Making a castor oil pack is pretty simple. There are convenient packs you can buy, which include a piece of wool. Or you can use an old T-shirt as follows:

1. Spread castor oil on your abdomen, taking care not to use too much; it shouldn't drip.
2. Place an old T-shirt across the oil.
3. Place a heating pad on top of the shirt.
4. Relax for 45–60 minutes.

5. Remove and wipe the remaining oil with the T-shirt or an old towel. Soap and water may be necessary if you feel too sticky, but most of the oil should be absorbed into your skin, or into the T-shirt.

It should be noted that castor oil is staining so old clothes should be worn when doing one. An old towel may be used if you don't want to risk staining what's underneath you.

Also, castor oil can cause skin irritation, so best to try it out on a patch of skin before applying it all over.

Do not wash the T-shirt afterwards. Castor oil is sticky and can leave a film in the washing machine. It is also flammable if you put it in the dryer. The T-shirt can be re-used a couple of times, but keep in mind that the whole process removes toxins, so it is best to use a new one as soon as possible.

There are different herbs— mustard seeds, fennel seed and turmeric—that can be added to the castor oil to increase the benefits as well.

Castor oil packs instigate a detoxification reaction in your body so the day(s) to follow you may feel some pain. With detoxification things feel worse before they get better.

With clear pathways, toxins are able to leave your body, helping decrease systemic inflammation.

SKIN: THE LARGEST DETOXIFICATION ORGAN

Another unfortunate side effect that came along with endometriosis and the related toxic overload in my body were annoying pimples on my face. As a woman in her thirties, I thought that I'd passed the period of breakouts. Wasn't that only supposed to happen to teenagers? I also struggled with painful eczema breakouts on my hands and fingertips for a long time. I recall coming home from work with gloves on my hands and tears in my eyes. The gloves protected my fingertips from having to touch anything directly. It hurt too badly.

Why was this happening to me?

As I dug deeper into researching a root cause for these skin issues, I learned that skin problems like eczema and dermatitis are generally caused by allergens exacerbated by toxins in our system. Our skin gives visible warning signs about our inner health and well-being. Often our outer skin is a reflection of our inner skin—our gut. Because of this, our skin is impacted by the food that we eat and toxic overload from the other things we come in contact with.

Dull skin and breakouts are signs that our inner detoxification channels are not working properly. When internal channels get clogged up, our body then attempts to release them out of our skin. Water, fat-soluble wastes, and gases are all released through the pores in our skin.

Another way that the skin gives signs of inner health is through sweat. The body odor that comes out is affected by the foods that we eat and the toxins we accumulate. I noticed this with my own smells when I ate something more toxic.

Skin absorbs everything we put on it, as well as the water that we bathe in. For this reason, I went by the advice to not put anything on my skin that I wouldn't put in my mouth. Instead of continuing to treat my eczema breakouts with a petroleum-based hand cream, I found relief with the help of coconut oil. But the creams and oils were only a temporary solution for a bigger toxic issue inside of my body that my skin brought attention to.

Our skin is actually the largest detoxification system in our body. To help support it, it is recommended to:

- drink plenty of water to cleanse and moisturize our skin;
- get enough sleep (our cells regenerate and repair during sleep);

- sweat out toxins with the help of exercise, sauna time, and/or steam baths;
- take epsom salt baths to help remove toxins through our skin (add a cup or two of epsom salts into a warm bath and soak for 15–20 minutes); and
- apply bentonite clay, which entices toxins out of your face, liver, feet, or wherever used.

The breakouts on my face and eczema breakouts on my hands and fingertips were eliminated as I moved along my healing journey and cleared up my detoxification channels.

Note: *When doing any kind of detoxification program, a short-lived break-out is very common, as large amounts of toxins are eliminated.*

THE LUNGS AND DETOXIFICATION

In his book, *The 3-Season Diet*, Dr. John Douillard goes deeper into another important detoxification channel: our lungs, which supply our blood with oxygen and extract toxins. In fact, our lungs dispense toxins with every exhalation.

Poor diet, air pollution, smoking, and shallow breathing may lessen the ability of our lungs to play their important role in the detoxification process. The contractions involved in our breathing help to transport lymph and blood to further dispel toxins. The lining of mucus and cilia—small hairs that capture airborne particles—found in our lungs help prevent toxins from entering our bodies.

How you breathe affects how you feel physically, mentally, and emotionally. Short, shallow breaths activate your sympathetic stress receptors, which catapult a variety of responses in your body that are no good for hormonal balance. Deep breathing of fresh air is the best exercise for our lungs. All it takes is 15 minutes of focused, deep breathing to make a difference.

Dr. Douillard explains how exercise is a great way to get the lungs moving, but while doing cardio, attention should still be kept on deep breathing to get the most out of the exercise and prevent the trigger of stress receptors.

Whenever I was feeling particularly toxic in my body or mind I shifted focus to activities that incorporated focused, deep breathing. I found yoga to be a great option for detoxification of my lungs, as focus is lent on deep breathing with movement.

In addition to exercise, another thing that helped was warm steam from a bath or shower, which was quick to moisturize my lungs and loosen up waste secretion. When I gave focus and love to my lungs through mindful awareness of my breath then a calming was initiated in my body. I could feel those toxins releasing already.

THE ROLE OF THE KIDNEYS

When I first started on my natural healing journey, I suffered greatly with bladder inflammation and pain. I took several trips to my primary care doctor sure that I had a UTI, but my tests continued to come back clean.

If it wasn't a UTI then what was causing all the truly aggravating pain in my bladder? With this question in mind, I continued my research and happened to come upon intriguing information from another Ayurvedic practitioner, Andreas Moritz.

His teachings lead me to believe that a lot of the pain and inflammation I was experiencing in my bladder related to the toxic load in my body and the subsequent impact on my kidneys. An unhealthy diet and unwholesome lifestyle can have a direct effect on our kidneys.

The kidneys are bean-shaped organs located on each side of your lower back. They are responsible for fluid and acid balance, metabolism, and elimination of toxins. When your kidneys get backed up with toxins kidney stones can form.

As mentioned, our kidneys are closely tied with our lymphatic system. The job of your kidneys is to release the final toxic byproducts. I found out that major diseases of the urinary system are caused by toxic blood as a result of lymph congestion.

Menstrual difficulties accompanied by lower back pain suggest kidney issues, as do bladder inflammation and pain. Another sign that your kidneys are stressed is the presence of dark circles under your eyes. I noticed this at times on myself and couldn't help but notice it on other people too.

KIDNEY CLEANSING HERBS

According to Dr. Moritz, the following herbs are designed to assist with detoxifying the kidneys:[15]

- Marjoram improves digestion and is an antiseptic, antibacterial, antifungal, and antiviral herb.
- Cat's claw stimulates the immune system and rids the body of harmful free radicals
- Comfrey root increases urination and aids in stomach disturbances.
- Fennel seed improves digestion and increases the flow of urine.
- Goldenrod treats urinary problems, bladder inflammation, and kidney stones.
- Gravel root treats urinary infections and kidney stones.
- Hydrangea root relieves bladder inflammation, kidney stones, and strengthens the urinary tract.
- Marshmallow root treats digestive disorders, anti-inflammatory.
- Uva ursi treats urinary tract infections, soothes, and strengthens irritated and inflamed tissues.

Present Moment (www.presentmoment.com) has created a kidney

tea with the above herbs to assist in flushing out toxins and sand from the all-precious kidneys.

Most issues that arise with our kidneys are related to an imbalance of the simple filtration system in our kidneys. The process of filtration is disrupted and weakened when our digestive system, and particularly our liver, performs poorly.

THE ALMIGHTY LIVER

In addition to its impact on our precious kidneys, I found that the health of your liver plays a huge role in the achievement of hormonal balance. This is because your liver is responsible for clearing out excess estrogen and aldosterone in your body. This is a big deal on the road to healing endometriosis.

The bile from your gallbladder stores these inactive hormones and excretes them, bound by fiber, in your stool. When gallstones congest in your gallbladder and liver's bile ducts, then estrogen and aldosterone are not sufficiently broken down and detoxified, so their concentrations travel back to your blood stream.

This leads to tissue swelling and water retention. Elevated levels of estrogen can also lead to abnormal cell growth including uterine fibroids, ovarian cysts, and endometriosis among other things. Elevated levels of aldosterone lead to muscle cramps, muscle weakness and tingling in your extremities.

When these unfiltered hormones travel back into your blood stream, then it is your lymph nodes' job to filter them out. This can lead to further congestion in your lymphatic system, which then leads to cysts in your uterus and ovaries, backaches, headaches, migraines, dizziness, thyroid enlargement, an enlarged spleen, and IBS.

The glands affected by congestion of your lymph nodes include your thyroid, parathyroid, adrenal cortex, and ovaries. When these glands are congested then a lack of hormones are secreted. This leads to, among other things, hypothyroidism and a negative impact on fertility.

Gallstones in your liver also cause liver cells to cut back on protein synthesis, which then prompts your adrenal glands to overproduce cortisol, a hormone that stimulates protein synthesis. Too much cortisol in your blood gives rise to a degeneration of your lymphoid tissue, leading to further blockages and a depressed immune system. In addition, an abundance of cortisol in your body leads to an accumulation of fat. This creates a problem since estrogen gathers in fat cells.

Added estrogens from the environment, including from birth control pills and HRT, increase bile cholesterol and decreases gallbladder contraction. This estrogen effect causes gallstones to form in your liver and gallbladder.

In addition to birth control and HRT, over-the-counter drugs and prescriptions are also damaging to your liver and contribute to gallstone formation. If your liver is weak and congested by these gallstones, then most nutrients pass through without being assimilated. So we can take loads of supplements to intake vitamins and minerals for years without effect. These supplements end up being waste products for your body to dispose of, causing even more work for your tired liver with little-to-no benefit.

Without a clean, efficient liver, blood is not filtered clean. This polluted blood is then loaded with hormones, toxins, and waste products rendering it heavier and more sluggish, leading to poor circulation. The result is constant fatigue, aches, and pains because the blood cannot efficiently carry needed oxygen and nutrients to the cells.

WAYS TO SUPPORT THE LIVER

The toxins that I collected in my body needed to be removed. This meant clearing up my detoxification channels. I focused much of my cleansing efforts on improving the functioning of my liver. I did a multitude of liver and gallbladder cleansing as outlined in Andreas Moritz's book, *The Liver and Gallbladder Miracle Cleanse.*

As I conducted these cleanses every couple of months I noticed a significant impact on my physical and mental well-being. The biggest impact came with a release of anger. In traditional Chinese medicine (TCM) it is believed that the liver is a storage depot for anger. As I released the years of toxins from my liver, I was met with a strong sense of calm, which was pretty foreign to me. Having a clearer head definitely helped me as I made a greater connection with the pain of endometriosis and the stress and anxiety in my life.

In addition to these cleanses, I found that there were plenty of other things I could do on a daily basis to help support liver functioning. One such thing was exercise. For me, this translated to morning yoga. Exercise helps to stimulate blood circulation. Early morning exercise that includes stretching and deep breathing exercises brings the blood out of your liver, which could be stagnant from its work the night before. Your liver does most of its work between 2:00–4:00 a.m. Drinking at least eight ounces of room temperature water right after waking up also helps move out the toxins that remain from your liver's nightly work.

Additionally, there are certain foods that boost's your liver's performance. According to Dr. Sandra Cabot's book, *The Liver Cleansing Diet*, the following are foods that support your almighty liver: [16]

- carrots
- cucumbers
- parsley
- cilantro

- celery
- green apples
- leafy greens
- beets
- garlic
- avocados
- lemons
- walnuts

Eating raw fruits and vegetables is helpful for your liver since raw foods contain more living enzymes that support digestion and assimilation. Juicing and/or smoothies are a great way to get in lots of raw fruits and vegetables. Your liver truly loves this.

GLUTATHIONE, THE ULTIMATE ANTIOXIDANT

As I looked deeper into ways to improve my liver I found that a significant component in improving liver functioning is glutathione, an important antioxidant. It's in every cell in your body, but in highest concentrations in your liver. Glutathione helps clean out toxins in your body from heavy metals, pesticides, solvents, and plastic residues like BPA. It also cleans up the end products from your body's metabolism called oxygen free radicals, which cause damage to cells. Glutathione disarms these oxygen molecules so they don't damage your body.

There was a study done that examined relationships between reactive oxygen free radicals that cause cellular damage and the growth of endometrial tissue in endometriosis.[17] This study found that endometrial cells have increased oxidative stress and have alterations in their detoxification pathways. This lends the suggestion that there could be a link between oxidative stress in your body and endometriosis.

Your body will have low glutathione levels if the body lacks the raw materials required for making it and with so much work to do, glutathione is always getting used up and constantly has to be made in your body.

Glutathione is composed of three amino acids: cysteine, glutamic acid, and glycine cysteine. To increase glutathione, it helps to increase intake of these three amino acids. Out of the three, cysteine is the most important because it contains sulfur, which binds to mercury. Food sources of cysteine include:

- poultry
- egg yolks
- red peppers
- garlic
- onion
- broccoli
- Brussels sprouts
- oats

Another way to increase glutathione is by supplementing with N-acetyl cystine (NAC). Research has shown that treatment with NAC helped reverse oxidative stress leading to endometriosis in mouse experiments and in vitro experiments.[18]

When glutathione levels are increased then your body starts to release all the accumulated toxins. This can cause a pretty severe detoxification effect. If supplementing with NAC, its best to start slow and take a low dose.

Another important mineral to keep glutathione levels high is alpha lipoic acid, the second most potent antioxidant. When glutathione does its job cleaning up free radicals it gets oxidized and is no longer able to clean up anything else. Alpha lipoic acid cleans up the glutathione and makes it ready to go back to work.

Food sources of alpha lipoic acid include dark leafy green vegetables, animal foods, and organ meats.

Glutathione is made by an important enzyme called glutathione S-transferase (GST). Both GST and another important enzyme called metylenenetrtahydrofolate (MTHFR) regulates detoxification pathways.

Many people have mutations in their genes that lead to a low efficiency of these enzymes in their bodies. In fact, most chronic illnesses are linked to a low efficiency of these genes. This is because with lower GST and MTHFR levels, glutathione levels get depleted very easily, which makes it harder for your body to remove toxins and heavy metals.

As we age, low GST and MTHFR levels can cause further havoc as your body accumulates more and more toxins and oxidative stress. Your body is then unable to replenish glutathione.

I found all of these discoveries about detoxification channels quite intriguing. As I continued to cleanse and feel better, this only prompted me to do further research. I felt like this was the true way for me to overcome the diseases that had taken hold in my body.

THE METHYLATION CYCLE

Further digging brought me to a grand discovery: the methylation cycle, which is central to our physical, emotional, and mental well-being.

The methylation cycle is part of the basic biochemistry of your body and is believed to operate in every cell. The methylation cycle performs many vital roles in your body including controlling your body's response to oxidative stress, which contributes to determining the rate of synthesis of glutathione.

When the methylation cycle is blocked, these important roles are not carried out properly. Two of the most significant effects of a methylation cycle block are that neither the immune system nor the detox system can operate properly. If the methylation cycle remains blocked for an extended period of time, infections and toxins can be expected to build up in the body.

If we have mutations in our genes that disrupt the methylation process then your body has a harder time releasing bad estrogens and endometriosis is fed. Enough mutations in this pathway lead to multi-factorial health issues including endometriosis and the autoimmune disease I'd developed, Hashimoto's.

MTHFR, THE GENETIC LINK TO ENDOMETRIOSIS?

In the methylation cycle, the methyleneterahydrofolate reductase (MTHFR) gene encodes the MTHFR enzyme. For some reason, scientists named both the gene and the enzyme MTHFR, which can cause confusion. But in short, a healthy, non-mutated MTHFR gene produced highly functioning MTHFR enzyme.

There are two main possible MTHFR mutations and we can have one or both. The specific mutation linked to endometriosis is MTH-FR C677T. This abnormality limits our ability to produce glutathione.

The MTHFR gene mutations, especially the C677T form, may also cause a deficiency in the body's largest carbon contributor, the chemical S-adenosylmethionine (SAMe), which is also very important for detoxification.

So what does this all mean for those of us with endometriosis? In order to process xenoestrogens, one must have functional detoxification pathways. If our genes are mutated or deleted then the elimination of these environmental estrogens is quite limited. This means that estrogen remains in your body as fuel for endometriosis. It also means that dioxins are unable to move out of our body. Studies have shown a link between dioxins and endometriosis.[19]

Mutated MTHFR genes can also be a causative factor behind multiple miscarriages. It is linked to chemical sensitivities, allergic responses, blood clots, anxiety, deep depression, thyroid issues, headaches, insomnia, fibromyalgia, and endometriosis.

The liver is very much involved in this process, including the turn of toxins to non-toxins so they can safely be removed from your body. When you drink alcohol, it is your liver's job to process it using methylation, but if nutrients are depleted or stress is in action, then your liver is not able to process the alcohol effectively. This leads to a hangover the next day. Genetic mutation of MTHFR means that your body has a much harder time detoxifying alcohol. This explained why I always felt so horrible after drinking alcohol.

Birth control impairs folate metabolism and is known to deplete folate. Therefore, if you take birth control and have the MTHFR C677T mutation, then levels of 5MTHF drop below normal, causing significant issues.

TESTING FOR MTHFR AND OTHER METHYLATION COMPONENTS

You may be able to get a blood test for MTHFR from your doctor or naturopath, but be aware that many times this is not covered by insurance. It depends on the health issue.

There is a company called 23andMe at www.23andme.com that sells self administered saliva tests to test for mutations in the methylation cycle. When the results come in from 23andMe then you can download the raw data file and run these results in different third party applications that help you decipher your genetic makeup.[iv]

It is important to know which kind of mutation, if any, you have before taking any supplementation.

---

iv   Genetic Genie (www.geneticgenie.org) For a donation, they run the 23andMe raw data into a report that will show a limited number of genes, including the MTHFR genes.

MTHFR Support (www.mthfrsupport.com/reports-consults/) For a small fee they run the 23andMe raw data and report over 100 gene results.

NutraHacker (www.nutrahacker.com) Provides a breakdown of your genetic mutations and what that means for your health. There is also a tool that helps determine that supplements to take and avoid, improving your individual genetic mutations.

It seems there is a growing awareness about methylation mutations that could be a key to earlier identification of potential health issues, including endometriosis. It is positive that there are steps in place to help with this deficiency.

Nutrigenetics is a relatively new field and much further exploration is needed. When I received my genetic results I realized that I'd opened up a big can of worms. It was a loud reminder that everything in the body truly is connected. Having this information provided a very individualized road map as to why my body developed diseases like endometriosis, while giving me a better idea of the further steps needed for healing.

I admit, at first I was overwhelmed with the multiple issues I found in my methylation cycle. However, I was aware of another emerging science called epigenetics, which includes the ability to change gene activity without changing gene sequence, meaning no mutations involved.

The study of epigenetics provides evidence that diet, lifestyle, and mental shifts can improve our genetic make-up. Epigenetics affects include the methylation process. This means that our genetics are not our destiny. We can alter how these processes by feeding our bodies healthy foods and reducing stress.

LESSON SIX: STRESS IS THE TRUMP CARD

"You must learn to let go. Release the stress. You were never in control anyway."

Steve Maraboli, Life, the Truth, and Being Free

To Achieve, to Please, to Stress!

The whole reducing stress thing was definitely a struggle for me. As a young woman I was prone to large amounts of stress in my life that more often than not related to a packed schedule that left very little time for fun or relaxation. Sleep was an afterthought to all that I needed to get done.

I was a type-A personality who was an over-achiever at heart. I liked to set goals. I liked the reaction I received when these were met. I loved to learn. I always wanted more. I strived to achieve high marks in school and to be at the top within my positions in my professional life. I was drawn to jobs in sales where my true competitive nature came out.

I enjoyed being at the top of the charts. When this didn't happen then stress and feelings of failure surfaced. This made me push harder. I liked control. This made it hard for me delegate tasks. It made me take on more than I should have. I struggled asking for help.

Other times my desire for perfection made me quit before I completed something if I felt like it wasn't up to my standards. This kept me from having to face criticism.

I worried too much about what others thought about me. I worried about being different. This oppression was developed from an early age when I struggled with bullying as a young girl. I grew up in a time of mandatory school busing where kids from the other side of town came to the elementary school close to my home. When it came to the color of our skin, I obviously stood out. My nickname soon became White Girl.

This was the first time I really recognized that I was different.

I struggled through the years of school that followed and recalled several instances where I avoided walking down a certain hall in my middle school, fearful of other girls that wanted to get out their aggression on me with their fists, or maybe just a good hair pulling. I couldn't understand why these girls wanted to fight me. But it definitely invoked stress in me at an early age, during the time when my hormonal development began.

The continued desire to want to be liked carried through my life, a quiet underlying thought that drove me to achieve. To please. With little consideration for how I was treating the key ingredient—me.

In retrospect I realized a lot of the drive to achieve and please came from a continued desire to find direction and ultimately worth in my life. In short, achievement and acceptance informed my perceptions of self-worth.

THE STRESS CONNECTION

By the time that I received my official diagnosis of endometriosis at 29 years old, I'd spent the previous 11 years working 40-plus hours a week, while attending undergraduate studies fulltime followed by graduate school part-time.

I was always studying or stressed about writing a paper or cramming for a test. Eleven years of higher education is a very long time. I really should be some sort of doctor by now. But by the end of it all I had two master's degrees under my belt, which was great. But in the meantime I'd managed to burn out my adrenals.

And I must say that the drive didn't stop with the collection of dusty diplomas somewhere in my closet. I was always—*always*—seeking more. I felt unproductive when I relaxed. It took me a long time to figure out the connection between the stress in my life and the health of my hormones; it turns out that stress throws everything off balance. This comes from the intricate interplay between the nervous and endocrine systems.

I learned about the important connection of these systems from Dr. Libby Weaver, a leading nutritional biochemist, author, and speaker who is passionate about women's health. She helped me bring attention to the two parts of my nervous system: the sympathetic nervous system (SNS) and parasympathetic system (PNS). These two systems are designed to balance each other out.

The PNS conducts processes that are out of our control like heart rate, respiration rate, temperature control, immune, and hormonal systems. The SNS is activated by stress and stimulates the body's stress hormones, which include adrenaline and cortisol.

THE ALL IMPORTANT ADRENALS + STRESS HORMONES

Our adrenals are part of our endocrine system, along with our pituitary gland, thyroid, parathyroid, and ovaries. Our adrenal glands sit at the top of our kidneys and are super important for balance and healing.

The outer part of our adrenals glands is called the adrenal cortex. This is where our hormones and pre-hormones are produced including:

- aldosterone, a hormone that regulates blood pressure
- dehydroepiandrosterone (DHEA), a pre-hormone for testosterone and estrogen that also regulates blood sugar and lipids
- adrenaline, designed to help our body escape danger or what it perceives to be dangerous
- cortisol, the stress hormone

Adrenaline communicates to every cell in your body that life is in danger. It is designed to help your body escape from pending danger and sends it into fight-or-flight mode. Adrenaline makes your heart race. It communicates to your liver and muscles that energy is required and converts glycogen into glucose and dumps this into your blood, thereby raising blood sugar levels.

When your body is in a near-constant state of red alert from psychological stressors, then life is lived in a state of tension. The blood supply to your digestive system is diverted to your arms and legs to prepare your body to get out of danger. Reproductive functions are downsized since they use a lot of energy and are not needed for immediate survival. Also, your body does not think it is safe to bring a baby into the world, so your adrenals stop producing progesterone.

Caffeine is a powerful drug that drives your adrenal glands to produce adrenaline. This puts your body in red alert. If hormone balance is your goal, it's time to say "no" to the coffee. This pains me even to write this. I love coffee.

With today's constant stressors, our adrenals are often in overdrive. When your body is under stress then your adrenal glands secrete high levels of cortisol and continue to do so until the stressor goes away. If the stress does not go away then eventually your adrenals tire out.

With sustained stress DHEA is the first of your adrenal hormones to get depleted. When DHEA levels are low then this is a sign that your adrenals are in trouble. Since DHEA is a precursor hormone, testosterone levels also drop. DHEA and testosterone support sex drive; maintain muscle mass and bone density. It also regulates cholesterol and blood sugar levels.

Patterns of tired adrenals include:
- waking up tired;
- feeling best in the middle of the day;
- crash and the need for a nap in the late afternoon; and
- second wind at night.

I don't know about you, but this pretty much summed me up.

IMPACTS OF EXCESS CORTISOL

The ever-present stress in my life triggered the release of the hormone cortisol. Since the stress had been present for a while, my body believed that there was imminent danger. This suggested to my body that it should hold onto body fat for survival. This is why the over presence of cortisol makes it hard to lose weight. And as mentioned previously, estrogen gathers in our fat cells.

If there is too much cortisol in your body then progesterone levels drop creating an environment of estrogen dominance. Without enough progesterone, the natural inclination is to overreact to things, especially leading up to menstruation when progesterone should peak.

According to Dr. Libby, some symptoms of low progesterone include low mood, unexplained weight gain, inability to lose weight, challenges conceiving, fluid retention, poor thyroid function, and anxiety. Progesterone is an anti-depressant and anti-anxiety agent, which is crucial for clear thinking.

If there is too much cortisol for too long then our adrenals slow down and eventually burn out. This starts with what has been termed as adrenal fatigue leading to adrenal burnout. At a burnout point, cortisol is negligible and fatigue is ever present.

Other signs of low cortisol include puffiness, stiffness, and achiness in your joints and muscles especially when cortisol levels should be at the highest. When your body has low cortisol it causes lower levels of the neurotransmitter norepinephrine, putting your body at a much higher risk for inflammation. Essentially your body is unable to control the immune system and unable to conquer inflammation.

Low functioning adrenal glands increases the risk of developing an autoimmune disease including thyroid diseases such as hypothyroidism, hyperthyroidism, Grave's disease, and Hashimoto's; rheumatoid arthritis; and lupus.

Low functioning adrenal glands can also be a causative factor in infertility. Ironically, infertility was one of the most stressful things I ever had to deal with, which only made things worse.

Everyday stress is going to happen. Life can get messy. It's really the long term, chronic stress that is most damaging. I encourage you to evaluate your own life and what's causing you chronic stress. Do you hate your job? How are your relationships? What part does spirituality play in your life?

If there is a long-term stressor in your life, what can you do to change this? If you are unable to change the stressor, then is it possible to change your reaction to it? By learning to have a different kind of response to a stressful situation, we avoid turning on the body's damaging stress hormones and save the health of the all-important adrenals.

BALANCING THE PARASYMPATHETIC NERVOUS SYSTEM

To help balance the interplay in your nervous system, it is important for your parasympathetic nervous system to be in line, as this is a major player in restorative practices in your body. Sleep allows your body to access the rest and repair part of the PNS. If we don't sleep enough then your PNS suffers. We should be getting a minimum of seven hours of sleep each night, but preferably eight or more.

Going to sleep at the same time and waking up at the same time sends a powerful message to your endocrine system. It is best to get to bed prior to 10:00 p.m. so your body takes advantage of the human growth hormones produced during this time, which are necessary for repairing your body.

Breathing is the cornerstone of adrenal support and the only way to consciously affect your PNS. Deep breathing should be a daily activity. It communicates to every cell in your body that you are safe and is most effective when done in a deep diaphragmatic way. In other words, makes sure your tummy moves in and out.

To keep your PNS happy, moderate exercise is important—not too much, not too little, Goldilocks. Rather than focus on high intensity exercise, sympathetic nervous system-dominant women should do gentle exercise like tai chi, qi gong, and restorative yoga— anything that focuses on your breath.

Note: If you are stressed out, or feel quite out of balance hormonally then higher intensity exercise only adds additional cortisol to the mix. This makes balance even harder to achieve.

Your breath is a powerful force that can naturally disrupt your nervous system, in a good way. As we've already seen, we also release toxins with deep breaths.

One simple breathing practice that you can incorporate into your life is an exercise that I learned about from Dr. Andrew Weil, an integrative doctor who is a strong promoter of this natural practice. The exercise includes a breath count of four-seven-eight that helps to lower stress, anxiety, and pain to leave your body in a relaxed state.

Basically you breathe in through the nose for four counts, hold it for seven counts, and then release it out of the mouth for eight counts. The tip of the tongue should set behind the back of the top two front teeth. This simple breathing exercise is great to incorporate when you fell stressed, anxious, like you're going to burst with unyielding negative emotion, wanting to double over in pain, or tossing and turning in bed.

RELEASING STRESS THROUGH THE PSOAS

The introduction of yoga into my routine truly changed my life and saved me from back surgery. Yoga helped me connect to the power of my breath, my life force, and helped me to release the stress in my muscles including an important one in relation to pelvic pain called the psoas (SEW-as) muscle.

Your psoas is one of the largest muscles in your body. It extends from your mid-back to the quadriceps and is the only muscle that connects your upper and lower body. It is one of the first muscles to develop in the womb, the core of development. The psoas has almost as many nerve endings as your brain. These nervous connections interact with your brain and nervous system. Its nerve endings also connect with your kidneys, heart, diaphragm and reproductive organs.

The psoas is the primary muscle that activates fight or flight. It instructs your nervous system to activate. By releasing and relaxing this massive muscle, you stimulate relaxation through your body and reduce both mental and physical stress. Loosening up the psoas can help hip and lower back pain.

In more extensive cases of endometriosis, your psoas can actually be inhibited by scar tissue. In this case, myofascial release can be helpful.

OTHER OPTIONS TO SUPPORT THE PNS

Another option that has helped keep my PNS in check is the practice of regular massages. There are many benefits to getting regular massages and healing endometriosis. One of which is getting your lymph moving to remove toxins from your body. Massages are also great for relaxing your body.

They forced me to slow down for at least an hour. Ha.

If your funds are too low to pay for regular massages, then self-massage can be helpful as well. Using a warm washcloth to massage into your skin can be relaxing. Another option is to use warm oil for your self-massage. Just be sure not to put oil soaked towels in the washing machine!

I found that a warm bath is also helpful for stress relief, especially with the addition of Epsom salts. Epsom salts contains magnesium and helps relax our muscles. This practice has helped me so much with the stress of out of control physical pain too.

To further support your PNS, it is important to have adequate protein and vegetables throughout the day, while limiting intake of white flour and sugar. We should also limit exposure to toxins and make time for relaxation each day.

I've found that expressing myself creatively really helps with stress too. When I am creative, other stressors drift away. It gives me a positive outlet and the opportunity to create something to enjoy later, a reminder of my thoughts and of a moment of inspiration.

CONNECTING WITH NATURE

I learned a lot about stress and hormonal imbalances from Ayurvedic practitioner, Dr. Claudia Welch in her book, *Balance Your Hormones, Balance Your Life*. She taught me the important connection of our bodies to nature through circadian rhythms, which control appetite, energy, mood, sleep, and libido. They also control timing quantity and quality of hormones and neurotransmitters.

Orderly rhythm is essential for optimal health. To find this order we turn to the divine teacher: nature.

Dr. Welch recommends a practice that can be really helpful to keep this rhythm in line: a walk outside everyday at the same time. The body needs to connect with the outside every day. I found walks outside to be very calming and a great active meditative practice.

The most important cue from nature is the sun. Our bodies should naturally rise with the sun and rest once it lowers. We should eat our biggest meal when the sun is highest in the sky, as this is when digestive juices are at their peak too.

Artificial, fluorescent lighting messes with our circadian rhythms by fooling the body with light outside of the sun.

All it takes is 15 minutes a day outside to soak in the healing powers of the sun and this living light in your cells to release stress and improve your immune system.

SHIFTING FOCUS TO ME

Within the journey of healing, I discovered that much of my stress came from my consistent desire to achieve. This drive produced the pursuit of a higher education and led to a corporate job where I strove for recognition. Along with this came a bunch of stress and not enough downtime for rejuvenation.

Self-care was an afterthought.

After reaching a point of exhaustion with a body that was breaking down, I finally discovered a critical missing piece. I'd seemingly forgotten about the most important person in my life: me.

Amidst all the chaos, I had to learn how to rest. Seriously. I had to remind myself that it was necessary. So, I unplugged. I took time for walks in nature. I started to read more, for fun. I took time for warm baths with essential oils. I cooked myself healthy foods. I fueled my soul by writing, everyday.

At last I reconnected with what I needed to feel well. Once I recognized my own requirements for self-care and became disciplined about making sure these were in place, my stress levels dropped significantly.

When I built self-care into my life then I was better equipped to truly enjoy this life.

This was not always easy. It entailed more use of the word *no*, something that was hard for me. But, I realized that if I didn't stand up for myself, then no one else was going to. I had to overcome the worries that I had about what others thought about me when I said that powerful two-letter word: no.

REQUIREMENTS FOR SELF CARE

If you are like me, then maybe you've never stopped to evaluate what *you* need. What makes you feel happy, content, relaxed, energized, at peace?

To help figure out your personal requirements for self-care, I found the following exercise from health guru Jennifer Louden to be very helpful:

Write out your answers to the following questions. Write whatever comes to mind for a minute or two; just keep your pen or fingers on the keyboard moving.

Questions:
1.) Without _____ I lose myself.
2.) When I feel most connected to my center I am _____.
3.) When I feel most connected to something larger than myself I am _____.
4.) I could live without _____ but not for long.

Look for consistencies in your answers. What do *you* need? Write these consistencies out and put them in a place where you will see them every day. Break them down into daily, weekly and monthly reminders and don't forget to check in.

Are you meeting your requirements?

When I met my requirements I felt much more grounded, balanced. I was finally caring for my body in more ways than just the food that I ate. At last I'd discovered the importance of disconnecting from all the messes outside and reconnecting inside, each and every day. Instead of worrying about what others thought about me, I turned my focus to improving what I thought about me. How was I treating myself? What words was I telling myself? How was I caring for *me*?

With this shift, magical things started to happen and the potential for true healing presented itself in a place deep inside that'd been unacknowledged for most of my life.

PEACE
WITH
ENDO

"Our suffering is holy if we embrace it and look deeply into it. If we don't, it isn't holy at all. We just drown in the ocean of our suffering."

~ Thich Nhat Hahn, Heart of the Buddha's Teaching

WHO AM I?

When my father posed the all-important question about my spirituality prior to my wedding day, I didn't have an answer. I didn't know how to define *what I was* in spiritual terms. But it stirred up a desire to find a response.

These questions were asked of me in a time of my life where I was experiencing chronic physical and mental struggles, preceding a tremendous shift in my life's direction and beliefs about myself.

Who am I?

So along with my studies about healing from a physical standpoint came examinations into true healing on a greater, spiritual level.

When I thought about spirituality's role in my life at the time, I suppose this gravitated most to my practice of yoga. Yoga truly changed my life. Because of this, I think I gravitated towards Eastern methodologies, which lead me naturally to the teachings of the Buddha.

As I learned more about the Buddha's life and his teachings, I became even more intrigued. He found a place of pure peace, of enlightenment underneath the Bodhi tree, a place free from pain.

This sounded good. I was drawn to meditation, to mindfulness, to simple principles of kindness, love, and karma.

Most of all, I was drawn to the Buddha's relation to the subject of suffering physically and mentally—a topic that, at the time, consumed much of life. I had a strong desire for this suffering to cease and I felt like his teachings laid a foundation that helped me figure out how to get there.

In the words of Thich Nhat Hahn in his book, *The Heart of the Buddha's Teaching*, "When something causes us to suffer, if we look deeply into it, we may see that it is exactly what we need to restore our happiness. In fact, suffering is essential for happiness."

This was a new way of thinking! I found that it very much related to the pain that I had endured from endometriosis. This force of suffering led me to examine what was causing the pain. What was causing the suffering in my body and mind?

SUFFERING AND SEPARATION OF THE TRUE SELF

Following the way of the Buddha helped me take a deeper step towards transformation as it helped me to identify the desires and effects clearly so I was able to stop the negative patterns I'd built over the years.

This direction was lead with the foundation of Buddha's Four Noble Truths:

- The First Noble Truth recognizes the presence of suffering of a physical and mental nature as a natural part of life. It also recognizes that there is a tremendous potential for joy and fulfillment.
- The Second Noble Truth follows with purpose in finding the cause of this suffering. Where does it originate?
- The Third Noble Truth seeks out the end of suffering. If there is no end, then what is the point? This Truth presents the belief that healing is possible.
- The Fourth Noble Truth lays out a road map to obtain true Nirvana.

Nirvana is a transcendent state in which there is no suffering, desire, nor sense of self. Some factors involved on the journey to Nirvana incorporate:

Right View: recognizing seeds of consciousness and watering these thoughts with wholesomeness. This piece includes the action of "waking up" and seeing things as they are. Most suffering comes from perception. By looking deeply into these perceptions, we can then be free of them.

Right Thinking: includes the "speech of the mind." These thoughts reflect our reality and the way that things are. Much of this thinking is unnecessary and causes undue stress.

Right Mindfulness: incorporates the action of being in the present moment. When we learn to live in the now then we are able to truly experience the glories of life and love.

This truth is better encompassed with conscious breathing that connects the body and mind – creating true wholeness.

FINDING TRUE LOVE

What about God? The existence of a higher power was not clear in my readings on Buddhism, but I couldn't break from the thought of some type of perfect higher power. I very much believed in a great, connecting entity made up of pure love. I believed that this love made up and connected every living thing. This was my true "religion."

I spoke to this perfect entity of pure love each day. I expressed my gratitude and prayed for safety and good health for my family and friends. I prayed for all the other women in the world struggling from the pain with endometriosis, from the pain of infertility and loss.

When my lips stopped praying, a sense of peace filled me. I had expressed my desires and thoughts to the universe and left the control for the outcome in the hands of love.

DEVELOPING A MEDITATION PRACTICE

While prayer was my way of speaking to God, I also spent time meditating. I heard meditation described as time spent listening to God, listening in golden silence.

It's been recognized that daily meditation significantly reduces stress and reduces cortisol levels in your body. Taking 10–15 minutes to meditate, sitting in silence with focus on your breath, has such a grounding effect. It is very calming.

I tried to get my meditation time in first thing in the morning, before the hustle and bustle of the day began. I tried different methods—sitting and focusing on my breath, counting my breath...but I struggled to control my "monkey brain."

I'd sit trying to find the silence, but quickly found that this was harder said than done. Many of my thoughts were on things that I needed to get done. Or random thoughts like, what was I going to eat later? Finding the silence was a struggle as was finding the now, where it was just me sitting there doing nothing. Could I just sit and be me? I got frustrated with myself and walked away from my attempted stillness feeling unfulfilled.

Would I ever be able to empty my mind?

Eventually the frustration I felt with my stirring thoughts taught me to become an observer of those thoughts. Instead of trying to push them away I acknowledged them—and *then* pushed them away.

The mind is a very powerful thing and within it are great healing capabilities and an even greater intuitive power. When I took the time to listen, in silent moments shared with myself, a deeper connection was made. Meditation and self-reflection helped me to stop and listen, to connect with the inner place where all the answers lie. The more that I listened, the more intuitive I became. The more balance in my life, the more synchronicities kept happening.

MINDFUL MEDITATION

My go-to meditation was a simple mindful meditation where the underlying point was to fall into my surroundings within the present moment.

The pull of nature allowed an easier transition to this mindful practice and an enjoyable one. The more time that I spent in nature, the more I was able to heal. I discovered that the power to heal and stay healthy is in the present moment, right now.

I started out with a simple mindful manner where the goal was to just sit, breathe, observe, feel, and acknowledge. I enjoyed this most when I could do this outside.

I rolled my toes through the cold grass and felt the sun on my knees. I took a long breath in of the warm air around me and closed my eyes.

My ears shifted to the sounds of the birds singing, of the sound of a lawnmower in the distance or an airplane flying overhead, the sound of the wind rustling through the trees.

When thoughts came to mind, I acknowledged them, and then let them pass. I turned my attention instead to that beautiful moment of simply being.

When I opened my eyes I took in the gorgeous green landscape around me. I experienced gratitude for the shaded canopy from the big trees that have stood on this earth likely longer than I.

Once I rose from these mindful meditations, I felt much calmer.

MEDITATIVE AFFIRMATIONS

I found another option for a simple meditation was with the use of meditative affirmations. Some examples of these include:

"I am perfection."

"I am healthy."

"I am strong."

One of my favorites: "My body is perfect."

With focus on this affirmation, I sat in silence and ran these words through the mind: *My body is perfect. My body is perfect. My body is perfect...*

The words flowed with my breath, and as time passed, I found that focusing on these messages helped to calm me down.

Regardless of the disease that riddled my insides and brought me days of darkness, despite that which threatened my body's ability to bear a child—my body is perfect.

With endometriosis, I think it is easy to think opposite thoughts of these: *I hate my body. I am not healthy. I am weak and tired.* With infertility those thoughts transpired to: *I am a failure. I am unworthy.*

When I focused on sweet meditative serenity of positive affirmations, I did feel better. These practices became a necessary part of my day. I needed to take this time for my mental health, for peace within.

By repeating positive messages over and over, as silent peace flows through, I believed eventually my body came to believe it.

Any thoughts against this message caused only more worry, more pain. And who needs that?

LEARNING HOW TO BE HERE NOW

Meditation helped me to extend mindful practices into my everyday life with further recognition of the power of the present moment—the touch, the warmth of Ryan's arms around me; the wiggle of my Boxer pups' butts as I walked into the door and their sheer love enveloping me in sloppy kisses.

Within the practice of mindfulness came the connection with life and freed me to truly experience happiness and joy.

Mindfulness taught me to embrace my feelings, especially the difficult ones like anger and suffering. When these feelings arose I recognized them as enjoyable, not so enjoyable, or mutual.

If they were not pleasant then I learned not to stuff them down, as I did in the past, but rather recognize them and acknowledge that my feelings were real, here, right now. With the recognition of these negative feelings, I released lingering suffering.

Mindful behaviors helped me get back in touch with my body, in recognition of how I was feeling, of the causes and effects different choices made on my pain levels.

Getting back in touch with my body caused me to care more for myself; I recognized when my choices resulted in pain. Once I started to feel better, I just wanted to feel even better and better. When I suffered through days of pain, I recognized it as such, and did my best to remain calm, while I cherished the days when I felt good. Most importantly, I learned that my innate nature, my inner light was unbound, unparalleled, immaculate—perfect.

Once I was able to recognize the pain as what it was I was able to shift my mind from it.

Once I was able to recognize that I am more than this pain and that I am more than what this painful body portrays, I was able to find a sense of peace.

Peace with Endo.

THE MORE YOU LISTEN, THE MORE YOU WILL HEAR.

The wise spiritual teacher Ram Dass said, "The quieter you become, the more you will hear." This seems self explanatory, but digging deeper on this thought brought up further revelations for me.

I grew up with parents who appreciated silence. They were both pretty introverted, a trait that was definitely passed down to me: quiet and self-reflecting. When most people meet me this is the common adjective that I hear to describe me: quiet.

Hearing this makes me somewhat uncomfortable. It puts a bit of pressure on me to speak up, something that I've never really been that good at. On the contrary, I listened instead, a factor that I believe is just as important as speaking. What value to the word that fails to be heard?

The more you listen, the more you will hear.

As I grew older and developed my own spirituality, I discovered the power of my individual silence. With a musician husband and two crazy Boxer pups, I struggled to find the silence sometimes.

This silence scarcity made me appreciate early mornings—the break of light in the new day, the rising sun. In these early mornings, in the stillness, I blended in, spending time in silence to just be, reconnecting to me.

When I was silent, I fell within. Thoughts arose. I witnessed them. Then let go.

Being in connection with this center helped reduce my stress, keeping me clear headed, connected. I think this stress connection reduced because I was listening to me.

As I studied and learned more and more about the interconnectivity of the systems in my body, I realized just how powerful my body's ability to heal really is. When something is wrong, out of balance, then my body lets me know about it.

This was evident to me upon my painful journey to an official endometriosis diagnosis. I knew that the pain signals indicated something was awry, even though every doctor that I saw told me that painful periods were normal. Looking back, I see how frustrating this process was, primarily because I felt like the doctors weren't listening to me!

As I learned to fall silent and connect with my inner self, I was better able to detect the messages of my inner wisdom. I came to believe that we all have an inner doctor inside of us, a guiding force that has the answers.

When things were out of balance in a physical sense, as in the food I was consuming, then my body told me so. Endometriosis was quick to flare when I chose the wrong foods for my body. When I stuck with nutrient rich foods then the pain stayed away.

I learned to detect lifestyle imbalances as well. Many times these issues came from outside stressors, whether it was financial concerns, increased time commitments, relationship woes, etc. But most of the pain, I believe came from emotional imbalances.

While I've definitely taken on the personality of a quiet introvert, this doesn't mean that my mind was silent. My thoughts were filled with much negativity—worries, anxiety, and the unyielding desire to be loved.

Learning to listen to my inner wisdom, or what I came to relate to as my soul, I uncovered issues stuck from years ago. This included beliefs I developed about myself; feelings of unworthiness and fear. What was missing most of all was an internal love.

So often I got caught up in doing, pursuing, and achieving. In the process, I lost connection with myself. I let my own love slip away in lieu of external, alternative motives. In the process I not only lost the connection with myself but also missed out on all the beauty around, external messages beckoning to me.

A great act of love is listening. How powerful this activity is to others and to ourselves? Validation of what's happening deep inside, outside of the noise.

What is the reflection of our soul? What is needed? What is here? The silence holds the answer.

OUT OF CONTROL

Control. It is an issue that has reigned over me for a long time. Not an external force as much as one that came from an inner place that felt out of control manifesting itself in this disease.

One thing I've struggled with endometriosis is the lack of control over the condition.

We are told with initial diagnosis of this chronic condition that there is no cure. That it will spread.

The fears related to this came up often on my healing journey, especially when pain or other out of the ordinary symptoms showed up. I couldn't help but think: Is it spreading? Is it getting worse? The only way to know the extent of endometriosis is to literally cut in and see—a painful, costly process.

I think the pain that comes with endometriosis both physically and emotionally, has in and of itself been a cause of fear for me. I've lived my life worrying about the arrival of my period, especially when it is possible arrival fell during a time when a big event was planned.

The worst pain came from the start of my period. Most of the time this felt like there was a sharp object stabbing my insides, as if someone took a knife into my vagina and continued to stab my uterus and ovaries.

The lack of control over this pain strangled my insides. This pain ripped through me, pain that could not be resolved with any available remedy. All that was left was a fetal position, heating pad and a chorus of moans that carried through from waking to sleep.

FINDING FORGIVENESS

I related this to my history of literal stabbings near this area of my body. This started with awkward teenage fingers and a not so consensual first sexual experience to the scrape of the metal wand with subsequent pap smears not to mention the warm up of the cold, yet daring vagina clamps, to the colposcopies where I was stabbed with things in long succession.

This collection of experiences built in my cells in my pelvic region and played out with each shedding of my uterus, as a reminder of those traumatic experiences.

As I moved forward on my healing journey, I realized just how important forgiveness is. So many people shy away from the idea of forgiveness, but I've been reminded often that forgiveness does not justify the act; instead it releases my burdens, leaving a place for whole healing.

I admit this was not easy. I worked through anger, especially in light of the fact my fertility could forever be compromised. I spent time falling victim to the stabbings in my pelvic region, pain from outside sources inflicted on me. Why me?

This anger did no good. It did not affect these outside forces, it only reflected inside of me, collecting in my cells as painful memories. In truth, this past cannot be changed, no matter how much mental anguish went towards it.

Instead, with focused thought and an open heart, I forgave. I forgave the man who had little regard for a young virgin, who in his own desires inflicted an unforgettable pain. I forgave the doctors who repeatedly picked and probed me, in search of a nonexistent cancer, causing additional pain with each period.

With focused intention I offered forgiveness to all that trauma that had collected in my lower chakras over the years. Once this forgiveness rang true, these past hurts were released. I no longer allowed them to control me.

True healing comes when we release the power of the wound to control our lives. This release comes with acceptance and forgiveness. Once this is done then we can find our true sense of self.

As the pain stabbed me during my menses, in similar ways as the past, I breathed in and out and forgave me body that caused me this pain. With loving care, I was patient with my body's healing process.

WITH ACCEPTANCE COMES PEACE

I picked up the habit of acknowledging a love for my body, especially my women bits that caused me so much pain. With drops of essential oils I spread small circles over my ovaries and uterus with focused love. Sometimes I even spoke aloud, "I love you."

I harbored acceptance for this disease endometriosis, this chronic condition that had made a big dent in my life. With acceptance came peace. As I let go of the desire to control something out of my control. I preferred instead to put that power into the realm of the divine, which in my mind is made of pure love.

I passed along this love to myself with understanding that there would be good and bad days. I extended gratitude with good days, when the pain stayed away or when my period came in a mild manner.

Healing happens in the space where damaging thoughts are out of the way, in the prime state of pure consciousness. This state encompasses a strong self-awareness with no judgment. When we let go of negative judgment, we allow our world to transform and we feel greater and greater trust.

In this prime space, negative thoughts still invade. But rather than trying to shove them away with forced positivity, I've found it better to allow them to pass with awareness and acceptance. No judgment.

When I tried to suppress or force negative thoughts out, the more they pushed back in. Instead, I learned to let the feelings flow through, knowing that these thoughts and emotions will pass.

The feelings and beliefs I hold about myself continue to be a reflection of the condition of my life. When things get stressful or seemingly out of my control, I've learned to turn within, for here is where the answers are.

By tuning into my internal guidance system, I found what was right for me and learned how to encode the methodology within. I know I am on the right track when I feel the center of my love, without judgment.

By loving myself, going inward and following my heart I was able to find true, eternal love and peace.

I believe that we are all a part of a higher realm of pure love and a piece of this divine love is within every single one of us, and within every living thing. There is a place inside where we are whole, apart from our conditions on the outside.

True healing is so much more than the physicality in front of me. My true spirit is so much more than the broken body that I live in. By re-centering and reengaging with this inner love allowed for true healing.

POWER OF SURRENDER

When things got out of control and the pain was unbearable, I learned about the power of surrender. With surrender, the pain and suffering loses its pull. When the pain is unbearable, there is little else to do but just fall into it.

I brought focus on the feeling of this pure agony. I felt all the messages and wishes this pain sought to show me with a steady breath and pure focus. I found that this focus, this surrender, lessened the pain. It lost its power over me.

Letting go of fear and surrendering is not an easy thing to do, but when it is miraculous things can happen. This state encompasses a strong self-awareness with no judgment.

The pain sent a reminder of how strong I really was and just how strong any woman with endometriosis really is. When I got through the pain, I proved that I would not be defeated. It is a reminder that if I could deal with this, I could deal with anything.

For this I am grateful. The pain from endometriosis forced me to explore a whole new realm of possibilities and discoveries into the power of the body to heal itself.

This suffering prompted me to seek out spiritual meaning in my life and a higher level of consciousness, where I was able to rise above the pain. In recognition of my true self, which is so much bigger than the shell of my physical body.

COMPONENTS
OF TRUE
HEALING

"You must find the place inside yourself where nothing is impossible."

~ Deepak Chopra

HELLO AGAIN AUNT FLOW

I recalled the first cycle when my period arrived with little to no pain. I was in the bathroom stall at work. When I spotted the swipe of red on the toilet paper, I braced myself for what was coming. I hated when flow showed up at work. I waited and waited but the pain didn't show. I made it through the workday in a bit of shock.

When I greeted Ryan at home I told him that I had started my period and he gave me a really odd look. After nine years together, he watched as I experienced the worst period pain on record. Where all color was stripped from my face and my body shook in horrible convulsions.

I walked to the kitchen and started to prepare dinner. His odd glances continued.

"Are you sure you started your period?" he asked.

I laughed as the thought had passed through my mind too. "Positive."

The changes that I'd made over the past three years with diet, cleansing, stress management, and spiritual awakening brought me to that place of near normalcy. I was functioning just fine on the first day of my period. Instead of being curled up in a ball of horrible pain, I'd made it through a workday and prepared a healthy dinner. While this definitely didn't happen overnight, it happened eventually. I'd arrived.

I gave Ryan a kiss on the cheek and we swapped smiles.

WHAT DO YOU BELIEVE?

When I was first diagnosed with endometriosis, I was told by my gynecologist and the surgeon who did my laparoscopy that it was an incurable disease. I was told that it was a chronic condition and would only continue to get worse. I couldn't imagine the pain getting worse. The possibility of this created a sense of hopelessness and sadness. And those negative beliefs activated stress in my body.

My official diagnosis of endometriosis sprung feelings of fear, anxiety, anger, frustration, resentment, and other negative emotions that surely triggered consistent stress responses in my body, making it really hard to heal and actually making things worse.

In her powerful book, *Mind over Medicine: Scientific Proof That You Can Heal Yourself*, Dr. Lissa Rankin describes your body as a self-healing organism that is constantly striving to return to homeostasis. She provides a book full of scientific proof that you can alter your body's physiology just by changing your mind.

Changing thoughts to those that are hopeful and optimistic can change how your brain communicates with the rest of your body and alters your biochemistry, setting the stage for your body to heal itself.

Within her personal practice Dr. Rankin notes that many of her patient's health conditions were cured by reducing stress, relaxing your body and mind, following a dream, and/or finding love. This positive flow induced physical, physiological changes. Many overcame the "incurable."

In her book, Dr. Rankin also writes a lot about following your internal guiding system. By realigning spiritually and reconnecting with this inner guidance your body becomes ripe for miracles. I believe that my healing journey really began when I shifted my mind from the negatives about endometriosis to the positives. This belief is an example of the power of mind over medicine.

I learned that much of the suffering in my mind comes from perception. A simple shift in perspective really helps to move forward. Rather than getting angry or bitter at the pain in my body I stopped and reconnected with it.

While I might not have been able to fully cure endometriosis, I did believe that I could heal. There is a difference. The dictionary definition of the word *heal* is "to become whole."

THE INNER MD

Instead of believing that doctors knew what was best for my body, I learned to diagnose my own root causes and apply my own prescriptions to change. When I learned to listen to the wisdom of my body, I found the answers that I needed. In turn, my mind shifted away from the dismal diagnosis of an incurable endometriosis and a life riddled with chronic pain. I realized that my body was screaming at me to pay attention to imbalances within. Once I took note and took action, I found that healing was possible.

While my periods did not remain completely pain free, they were a vast improvement from where I once was. I was able to function and carry out the daily tasks that were required of me. When things did get painful, I took this as a reminder from my body that I needed to slow down and rest. The pain brought attention back to my inner MD who was quick to ask questions.

- What was causing the pain?
- Was there something that I did; something that I could avoid in the future?
- Was I stressed?
- Was I sleeping enough?
- Did I need to slow down?
- Eat better?

With time I learned how to care for myself as arguably my own personal best doctor simply by listening and reconnecting to my body. Endometriosis made me stop and pay attention. It made me investigate my own life. It took some digging but I was able to uncover much of my root causes for this illness.

The digestive distress that had caused countless issues over the years like bloating, flatulence, and constipation nearly were non-existent. The daily headaches I had over the years were few and far between. I no longer needed pain pills or over-the-counter NSAIDs to get through the day. In fact, I arrived at a point where I no longer took them at all. I was reminded of this fact when others came over asking for them and I didn't have any in the house.

Best of all the angry, depressed, lost woman I once knew transformed into a positive, peaceful being with pure love and hope. This beautiful shift made me want to share this message with you.

You can find peace with endometriosis too.

The body has an amazing capacity to heal when given the proper nourishment. I wasn't feeding myself with good things in a physical or emotional sense. Once I started to pay attention to my choices and their impacts on my health, things shifted. Once I took action to release the toxins in my body and mind through regular liver cleansing, then real changes started to happen. When I released the physical toxins then it was easier for my mind to find peace and calm.

I believed that I could heal from this disease. I didn't need a doctor to tell me this. I needed to write my own prescription. If your mind is clear that there is no hope, then this sends a signal to your body that it is sick and will never get better.

Instead of spending my time around the general medical community, which was quick to spout out negative shortcomings of endometriosis and how it was incurable, I built a team of people in alternative wellness arenas who believed in addressing issues of health from a whole-body perspective with belief that endometriosis was an imbalance on the body that needed to be addressed as a systemic issue.

I found alternative methods of whole-body healing through Ayurveda, traditional Chinese medicine, functional and integrative medicines. For this I am thankful. I understood that I was not going to be able to figure this out all on my own.

I most definitely would not be where I am at today without the support of fellow endo sisters. To further aid in your individual healing, I encourage you to reach out to support groups. Reaching out improves feelings of isolation often related with endometriosis, which is a condition whose depths are not fully realized by those without it. There is nothing greater than connecting with other women who understand. I started a private, positive space on Facebook called "Finding Peace With Endo". I would love for you to join us there.

POWER OF INTENTION

The power of the words that follow *I am* are extremely important, for we become what we believe about ourselves. A big step to healing comes from the belief that we *can* get better. Once this intention was solid in place for me, I aspired to make it happen.

Scientific experiments outlined in the book, *The Intention Experiment* by Lynne McTaggert, show evidence of clear and focused intentions as being a catalyst for different physical changes. The message in this intriguing book is the scientific interconnectivity of living things to each other as messengers of energy. Scientific evidence suggests that for an intention to have significant impact different factors need to be in place including time, place, a quiet mind, visualization practices, and a strong belief that the intention will come true. Start with reasonable goals within a realistic time frame, while keeping a grand scheme in mind to build towards. For me, my grand scheme was healing from endometriosis, while I set smaller intentions along the way to help get me to this place.

In her book, Lynne suggests that your mind "power up" prior to setting a clear intention. This should be done in a comfortable, consistent space, away from electronics and other sources of outside energy, preferably in a place outside or where clean air is present.

In order to power up to a mental place where intentions manifest, your brain must first slow down its waves to a meditative state. Within your comfortable place, sit and relax your body and try and clear your mind. It is helpful to find an anchor—a connection with your breath, a mantra, numbers, or music such as chanting or a steady drum beat—that can help you reach the place of peace. Lynn recommends practicing your hold to this anchor until you can sit for 20 minutes or more.

This meditative state should be free from judgment with attendance to the present moment without preference for pleasant or unpleasant experiences. Each experience should be identified simply as something happening.

Once achieving this ideal mental situation, then clearly state your intention. Make sure it has an end point as a wish that has already been achieved. Evidence shows that specific intentions work best. Those that are highly specific and directed are more likely to happen. Include what you want to change and to whom, when, where.

Visualize the outcome you desire with all five of your senses in place. In achievement of this intention how would you feel? Imagine this feeling in your body. See the impacts this change will have on your life and those around you.

This intention could be a change in a stressful living situation, job, relationships, physical conditions or a state of mind (from positive to negative).

With endometriosis, this intention could be a life with no more pain. How would this feel? Imagine your body as agile, electrically alive, and free from pain. How did you feel before the pain of endometriosis came into your life? Be sure to include all sensations that support this healing process.

Visualizations could include a good vs. evil battle where the bad are endometrial implants or pockets of pain. Imagine these displaced cells changing into healthy cells. If you are in pain, then visualize the nerve endings in your entire body and "see" healing energy that enters with every breath.

Lynn suggests sending out this intention often during meditation and throughout the day. To help visualize the outcome of your intention, create a visual collage of what your end result looks like, perhaps images of what healthy and whole means to you.

Do not allow yourself to think of failure or dismiss your intention as not possible. It is less likely to happen when these thoughts are in place. And only send intentions when you feel happy and well to prevent negative thinking to creep in.

Once your intention is stated clearly, then the final step is to let go. Sense that it is taken over by a greater force. Take it as a request to the universe. I believe that focused intention really assisted me on my journey to healing. Once I put clear intentions in place, amazing things started to happen that impacted my life in very positive ways.

The days of chronic pain are behind me. This came with a lot of dedication and a belief that I could feel better. It came from taking action outside the box with a willingness to try new things and stand up for my health and well-being. It came from a clear visual of a life free from pain.

This is not to say that I don't still get bad days, especially with the start of my period, but I learned to shift my negative attitude towards it. After suffering countless painful periods, I think it was normal for me to dread the arrival of flow. Suffering with endometriosis made me *hate* flow. How could I not?

When Aunt Flow visited and I was able to function, this was an extreme victory. I learned to appreciate my period as a time to rest and recharge, as a time for self-reflection. Each cycle was a new beginning. This process of rejuvenation each month became an analogy for growth and renewal.

I LOVE YOU

Above all else, a key part of healing came from making time for self-care and a dedication to improving my inner beliefs that were conditioned from a very young age. As a girl, I took the mean words of other kids to heart. When I grew into an awkward pre-teen, I let the opinions of boys and mean girls take precedence in my mind. By the time I hit high school I had developed significant self-esteem issues. I wanted to disconnect from my reality. I was unhappy and just didn't care.

Looking back on those times makes me flinch. I was so disconnected from my body. That and lack of self-esteem related to a lack of self-love. I never learned to love myself. Perhaps I failed to ever really be lifted up. Things really changed for me when I made the decision to stand up for myself, because I wanted to feel better. I finally realized that I was worth it. Period.

Feeding my body with junk food was a betrayal. It was hurting my soul. My relation with food, drugs, and alcohol was a way of compensating something missing inside. I had no other relationship with food outside of the fact that it tasted good. Stopping to consider what I was eating—and why—made all the difference.

Another big turning point came when I realized I was restricting myself from different things not because I couldn't have them; I didn't want them because of the negative ways they made me feel. This mental shift made it easier to stick to healthy choices that were good for my body and mind.

I recognize that self-love is difficult with endometriosis. Loving a body that radiates pain is not always easy. I know that many times I thought how much I hated the body I'd been given.

These thoughts come more on pain days, or days where the struggle with infertility rose, or on those crazy emotional days where my inner wisdom cried out for attention. But as I healed and the daily aches and pains lessened my attitude improved, helping to keep the dark thoughts at bay.

Traveling all this way on my healing journey I've come to believe that self-love is the key to healing endometriosis. I wanted to feel better for me. I am worth it. I deserve to feel good. I deserve what is best for my body, what is best for my mind, and what is best for my soul.

I have learned many lessons on the continual road to self-love. I know now that this life is truly a gift. This is evident when I stopped for just a moment and looked around at the wonders of this world: the simple yet complex systems in nature; the wonders of the human body and its natural ability to heal; the wonders of new life; and the discoveries and animation of movement and spirit.

The body is the gateway to our human experience, a vehicle for our souls. We must take care of it. We must feed it with the best food and nutrients that we can. We must nurture it with rest and eliminate physical stressors. We must take time for ourselves to explore creative paths, to find laughter and contentment, to find peace.

FINAL THOUGHTS ON FERTILITY

I so wanted to end this collection of lessons with news that I was pregnant or that I have a child. This, however, is not the case. In retrospect, there was a greater goal that was met: I love myself anyway.

I know that one day Ryan and I will grow our family, whether or not it is in a traditional manner with natural pregnancy or in an alternative way like adoption remains to be seen. Either way, I have made acceptance with my body. All that matters is the present moment. No need to worry about what might, or might not, happen.

Between these spaces of time I am blessed with two beautiful boxer pups, my best friend, Ryan, and a much bigger unspoken love.

THE GREATEST LOVE OF ALL

When I fell upon dark days in the past, recurring thoughts resonated in my mind: *Nobody loves me. I am alone. No one cares.* This deep feeling of being alone and unloved sent hurt right to my heart, to my soul existence. Isn't the whole purpose of life to love and be loved?

I realized that during these times when I felt like I was truly alone, that no one cared, that my life was not worth anything, that I was wrong—very wrong. No matter how bad things got, there was always hope because ultimately there is a divine entity or energy that loves me and you; something that understands at a much deeper level.

After losing Jeff early in my adult life, I had so many questions. While his life was gone, I still felt his love. I still felt his presence. Where does this go after death? What happens? Intrigued by these questions, I started to read different stories of near-death experiences, of people who've come closer than most to what happens after death.

I found that these near-death recollections were similar. They included encounters with an energy source that is overflowing with love that is immediately recognized even in an existence outside of the human body. These experiences created notions that none of us are ever unloved. Every living thing is deeply known and cared for by a source that loves and cherishes us. This unspoken love is always there, even though it is silent.

I think that in order to recognize and truly feel this love, we must fall silent too. For when we take time to reconnect, we can feel this love deep inside. This love is unyielding. This love is enough.

Have you stopped to listen?

There is something more, a divine love that is everlasting, that understands each of us, that understands our pain and our struggles really helps when times are tough. This silent love is always there. Perhaps at times, we must fall silent and step outside our broken shells to really experience it.

AFTERWARD

The journey of life can be long and uncertain and fear is going to arise. Dark clouds will threaten to cover you and may rain down on you causing anxiety and stress, but as soon as you turn the corner you will be surrounded with light.

On a walk through the woods I spotted rows of bent aspens, golden, curved canopies that continued to grab my attention. These trees were in the shade, but bending towards the place where the sun hits. Another subtle cue from nature—sunshine is essential to life. Move towards the light.

It's so important to trust the inner intuition that inherently directs us down the right path. It is easy to ignore it or reason against it, but the message and direction is always there. Bat back at the fear and doubt and just keep moving. That is all you can do: put one foot in front of the other. Everything always works out.

Everything is connected. A big circle. No matter our doubts, we were on the right path the whole time. Nature teaches us this in a magnificent way. The sun and water nourishes the earth, providing food to us and energy to the forest of trees providing oxygen and a trail of life, connecting natural energy to our bodies and mind.

Any question on healing the body should go back to nature, for there the answers are presented. Cut out the unnatural. Put in that from nature, that with true energy and life, for that substance is healing.

But remember, nature is not quick. If you plant a seed in a ground today it will not be fully bloomed tomorrow. It takes time. It takes patience.

Thank you for sharing this journey with me. Sending you love.

CONNECT WITH AUBREE

Aubree's passion for health and wellness led her to becoming a certified holistic health coach. She supports women with endometriosis who want to manage their pain through natural methods including diet, lifestyle, and positive thinking.

Aubree offers one-on-one and group-coaching programs aimed at transforming your life through small, manageable changes. She creates a positive, motivating environment to help you reach a place of less pain, more energy, and a life filled with positive rhythms.

Aubree is also available for speaking engagements on nutrition, healthy lifestyle, stress management, and overcoming suffering.

To connect with her further please visit www.peacewithendo.com

REFERENCES

1   Center Disease Control and Prevention. Genital HPV Infection Fact Sheet. [Online]. Available: http://www.cdc.gov/std/hpv/stdfact-hpv.htm [2014, 9/13/14].

2   Cleveland Clinic. Facts About Endometriosis. [Online]. Available: http://my.clevelandclinic.org/disorders/endometriosis/hic_facts_about_endometriosis.aspx [2014, 9/13/14].

3   Northrup, Christine. (2010). Women's Bodies, Women's Wisdom. New York: Bantam Books.

4   Department of Nutrition, Harvard School of Public Health. (2007 February 18). Dietary glycemic load, whole grains and systemic inflammation in diabetes the epidemiological evidence. PubMed [Online]. Available: http://www.ncbi.nlm.nih.gov/pubmed/17218824 [2014, 9/13/14].

5   Ermakova, Irina. Influence of genetically modified soya on the birth-weight and survival of rat pups. [Online]. Available: http://somloquesembrem.org/wp-content/uploads/2013/01/Ermakovasoja.pdf

6   Ermakova, Irina. Influence of genetically modified soya on the birth-weight and survival of rat pups. [Online]. Available: http://somloquesembrem.org/wp-content/uploads/2013/01/Ermakovasoja.pdf

7   Bloom, Susan. (2013). The Immune System Recovery Plan. New York: Scribner.

8   Bloom, Susan. (2013). The Immune System Recovery Plan. New York: Scribner.

9   Moritz, Andreas. (2007). The Liver and Gallbladder Miracle Cleanse. California: Ulysses Press.

10   Douillard, John. (2007). The 3-Season Diet: Eat the Way Nature Intended. New York:Harmony.

11   Douillard, John. (2007). The 3-Season Diet: Eat the Way Nature Intended. New York:Harmony.

12   Lee, John. (2006). Hormone Balance Made Simple: The Essential How-to Guide to Symptoms, Dosage, Timing, and More. New York: Grand Central Life and Style.

13   Northrup, Christine. (2010). Women's Bodies, Women's Wisdom. New York: Bantam Books.

14   Douillard, John. (2007). The 3-Season Diet: Eat the Way Nature Intended. New York: Harmony.

15   Moritz, Andreas. (2007). The Liver and Gallbladder Miracle Cleanse. California: Ulysses Press.

16   Sandra Cabot The Liver Cleansing Diet

17   Faculté de Médecine, Service de Gynécologie Obstétrique II et Médecine de la Reproduction, AP-HP Hôpital Cochin. (2009 July). Reactive oxygen
species Controls endometriosis progression. PubMed [Online]. Available: http://
www.ncbi.nlm.nih.gov/pubmed/19498006 [2014, 9/13/14].

18   Faculté de Médecine, Service de Gynécologie Obstétrique II et Médecine de la Reproduction, AP-HP Hôpital Cochin. (2009 July). Reactive oxygen
species Controls endometriosis progression. PubMed [Online]. Available: http://
www.ncbi.nlm.nih.gov/pubmed/19498006 [2014, 9/13/14].

19   Department of Obstetrics and Gynecology, Vanderbuilt University
School of Medicine. (2002 August). Environmental Dioxins and Endometriosis.
PubMed [Online] Available: http://toxsci.oxfordjournals.org/content/70/2/161.full
[2014, 9/13/14].

32934051R00101

Made in the USAMade in the USA
San Bernardino, CA
19 April 2016